Clinical and
Oral Microbiology

Clinical and Oral Microbiology

PHILIP W. ROSS
TD MD ChB MRCPath MIBiol FLS

Senior Lecturer in Bacteriology
University of Edinburgh
Honorary Consultant Bacteriologist
Royal Infirmary Edinburgh

AND

W. PETER HOLBROOK
BDS PhD FDS MRCPath

Senior Lecturer in Microbiology
Faculty of Odontology
University of Iceland

BLACKWELL SCIENTIFIC PUBLICATIONS
OXFORD · LONDON · EDINBURGH
BOSTON · PALO ALTO · MELBOURNE

© 1984 by Blackwell Scientific Publications
Editorial Offices:
Osney Mead, Oxford, OX2 0EL
8 John Street, London, WC1N 2ES
9 Forrest Road, Edinburgh, EH1 2QH
52 Beacon Street, Boston,
  Massachusetts 02108, USA
706 Cowper Street, Palo Alto
  California 94301, USA
99 Barry Street, Carlton, Victoria 3053, Australia

First published 1984

Typeset by Scottish Studios and Engravers Ltd.,
Glasgow
Printed and bound in Great Britain by
Butler & Tanner Ltd.,
Frome and London

DISTRIBUTORS

USA
  Blackwell Mosby Book Distributors
  11830 Westline Industrial Drive
  St. Louis, Missouri, 63141

Canada
  Blackwell Mosby Book Distributors
  120 Melford Drive, Scarborough
  Ontario, M1B 2X4

Australia
  Blackwell Scientific Book Distributors
  31 Advantage Road, Highett
  Victoria 3190

British Library
Cataloguing in Publication Data

Ross, Philip W.
  Clinical and oral microbiology.
  1. Mouth—Microbiology
  I. Title   II. Holbrook, W. Peter
  616'.01'0246176   QR47
ISBN 0–632–01147–5

Contents

Preface

This book is intended to provide dental students with the fundamental principles of microbiology as they are applied to medicine and dentistry. It deals with infection of the body systems rather than the relation of individual organisms to particular diseases. The rapidly developing field of oral microbiology is introduced and this is intended to provide an academic background to clinical work. It is hoped that the book will prove useful to undergraduates, practitioners and to postgraduate students.

Students of dentistry should be aware of the role of microorganisms in the aetiology of dental caries and periodontal disease; they should be familiar with the nature and development of dental plaque and the normal oral flora. The causes and treatment of infections of the mouth should be appreciated as well as the hazards of cross-infection in dentistry, and there is also a need to be familiar with aseptic techniques and methods of sterilisation and disinfection as applied to dentistry.

Acknowledgements

We wish to record our sincere thanks to the following: Dr Helga M. Ögmundsdóttir for contributions to the text and for helpful advice; to the Medical Illustration Departments of the University of Edinburgh and the University Hospital, Reykjavík; to Mr Grétar B. Sigurdsson for many of the diagrams; to Dr Hallgrímur Benediktsson for helping to prepare several photomicrographs; to Dr Helga M. Ögmundsdóttir and Mrs Stella J. Ross for reading the proofs; to Dr R. Warren for compiling the index and to Mrs V. McGrath and Mrs M. Cole for typing the text.

CHAPTER 1

Introduction and History

The science of microbiology has shed much light on the nature of disease. In the nineteenth century the work of Pasteur, Lister and Koch did much to help explain the role of bacteria in disease and to indicate possible methods of practising safer medicine.

Louis Pasteur (1822–95) was the first scientist to show clearly that bacteria and moulds never generate spontaneously and that no growth of any kind occurs in sterilised media when precautions are taken to separate organisms from the surrounding air. One of his many achievements was the development of the technique of controlled heating known as 'pasteurisation' for the preservation of beverages and foodstuffs. Despite his discoveries in the field of science it was nevertheless the relevance of his work to medicine that set him apart as one of the most distinguished figures in microbiology. By his experimental studies on anthrax in 1876–77, for example, he was to prove that a certain type of infection invariably occurred when a number of microorganisms of a particular kind were introduced to the body. The cause-and-effect relationship was proved by showing that anthrax bacilli, made to multiply for many generations outside the body in serum and broth, retained their ability to cause in animals the particular infection with which they had been associated originally.

Joseph Lister (1827–1912) did most of his pioneer work on antiseptic methods in surgery when he was Professor of Surgery at the University of Glasgow (1860–69) and Professor of Clinical Surgery at the University of Edinburgh (1869–77). He was familiar with Pasteur's work on the presence of bacteria in the air and on their biochemical activities and postulated that the postoperative infections encountered so commonly in surgical practice could be explained by microbes present in the air and surroundings gaining access to the wound, causing 'putrefaction' and 'sepsis'. He, therefore, made it his practice to spray solutions of phenol around his patients and to use gauze dressings impregnated with phenol to cover the wounds. By doing so, although being unaware of the microbial causes which he was dealing, he transformed the face of surgery by reducing greatly the incidence of postoperative sepsis.

Robert Koch (1843–1910) was undoubtedly one of the greatest figures in the development of microbiology. Starting off life as a country general practitioner in eastern Germany he later turned his attention to bacteriology and problems of infection. He had immense skill in devising new bacteriological techniques; for example, he used aniline dyes to stain bacteria long before the method of Christian Gram was described in 1884. Methylene blue was applied to a dried smear on a glass slide which was then fixed and kept as a permanent record. He was also the first to make photomicrographs of stained smears, and in addition he pioneered methods of growing bacteria on agar media.

Unknown to each other Pasteur and Koch simultaneously investigated the cause of anthrax, during 1876–77. They both demonstrated its aetiology, and as a consequence the concept of the germ theory of disease was established. Koch was also responsible for describing the criteria that would determine whether a microorganism has a causative relationship with a disease (Koch–Henle postulates, p. 56).

Despite the fact that the germ theory of disease had been established in 1877 it was not universally accepted until 1882 when Koch presented his masterly paper on 'The aetiology of tuberculosis', giving details of the isolation of the tubercle bacillus.

1

In the following year he isolated the cholera vibrio.

The 'Golden era' of medical microbiology which was opened by Pasteur, Lister and Koch was perhaps the greatest single contribution ever to the theory and practice of medicine. In the first half of this century the role of viruses in disease began to be understood. In the last 40 years great developments have been made in antimicrobial chemotherapy and most recently man has begun to understand the host response to infection and to other material of 'foreign' origin. Immunology has thus grown into one of the most rapidly developing areas in the pathological sciences.

Development of microbiology in dentistry

In recent years there has been an upsurge of interest in the microbiological aspects of dentistry. First came the realisation that dental caries was caused by bacterial fermentation of sucrose with the consequent acid production causing the lesion. Periodontal disease was later found to have many links with dental plaque, the bacterial deposit that forms on the teeth in the absence of oral hygiene. The nature of dental plaque and the flora of the mouth was further investigated when improved techniques for isolating and culturing anaerobic bacteria became available.

As the result of much research a greater understanding of the relationship between man and his commensal flora is now emerging and this is of considerable help in elucidating the role of these microorganisms in disease. (Many of the mechanisms of bacterial interaction with host tissues such as adherence are often studied using oral organisms).

Clinical dentistry has developed in many ways in the last decade particularly in oral medicine and in this area microbiology has played a part in the understanding of mucosal infection and of the oral manifestations of systemic disease. Several developments in the field of antimicrobial drugs also have relevance to clinical dental practice and the dental practitioner now has to be familiar with a far wider range of these agents than hitherto.

It is salutary to realise that microorganisms in the human mouth were among the first to be described, by Antonie van Leeuwenhoek, as long ago as 1683. His astute observations on scrapings from carious cavities in teeth were made with the use of only a single-lens microscope, but despite such limitations he was able to describe the principle shapes of bacteria that remain the basis for much of the classification of microorganisms today.

In 1890 Willoughby Dayton Miller, an American chemist turned dentist, working in Berlin published a thorough and authoritative account of the microorganisms of the human mouth. It is to Miller that the credit usually goes for advancing the theory of the bacterial fermentation of sugar as the cause of dental caries. Miller himself gives credit to Milles and Underwood but there is no doubt that it was he who had the foresight to realise the implications of the earlier work and relate this to caries (Fig. 1.1). His

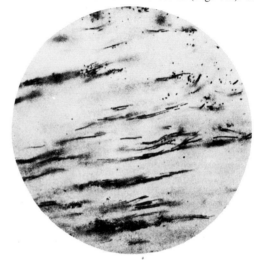

FIG. 1.1. Photomicrograph taken by Miller to show bacteria in dentinal tubules (courtesy of S. Karger AG, Basel).

conclusions about the involvement of dental plaque in periodontal disease are often regarded as less than astute but in many other ways the conclusions from his painstaking observations are still accepted today.

It is unfortunate that this early work was neglected for so long and that the aetiology of caries required rediscovery many years later. Even in 1965 a substantial review in the *Annals of the New York Academy of Science* on the mechanisms of dental caries only hinted briefly at the possible role of certain specific microorganisms in dental decay. Miller, however, stated in 1890 that 'the species of bacteria which possesses the highest ferment activity and the highest peptonising power and is able to flourish with a limited supply of air will, *caeteris paribus*, cause a more rapid destruction of tooth substance than another having these qualities to a minor degree .

FURTHER READING

Annals of the New York Academy of Science (1965) Mechanisms of dental caries. **131**, 685–930.

Miller W.D. (1890) *The Microorganisms of the Human Mouth*. Philadelphia: The SS White Dental Manufacturing Company. (Reprinted in facsimile (1973). Basel: S. Karger).

CHAPTER 2

Classification of Microorganisms

Microorganisms of medical and dental importance can be divided into several large groups including bacteria, viruses, fungi and a number of organisms intermediate between bacteria and viruses. Bacteria and these intermediate organisms are known as prokaryotes. Fungi together with some algae, moulds and protozoa with a more highly developed cell organization, such as is found in animals and plants, are eukaryotes. The principal differences between eukaryotes and prokaryotes are as follows:

Nuclear membrane
Nucleolus   *Eukaryotes* possess
Membrane-bound   *Prokaryotes* do not possess
mitochondria

Viruses are different from all other forms of life and do not fit readily into any larger groups.

Classification of bacteria

From the earliest studies of bacteria attempts have been made to classify the organisms; this has often been on the basis of shape which still forms the fundamental aspect of the accepted classification. A bacterium may be: spherical (a coccus), rod-shaped (a bacillus), comma-shaped (vibrio), spindle-like (fusiform), or spiral (spirillum). A branching filamentous form is seen in the so-called higher bacteria (Actinomycetales). Further groups are described usually on the basis of the arrangement of cocci into pairs (diplococci), clusters (staphylococci) or chains (streptococci) (Fig. 2.1).

In 1884 Gram described a staining technique that enabled bacteria to be seen clearly down a microscope and this observation divided the bacteria into two groups. Gram-positive bacteria appear blue-black because they retain the first two stains of the

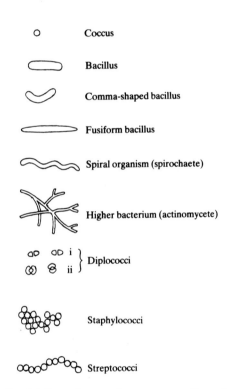

FIG. 2.1. Some shapes and arrangements of bacteria.

technique, crystal violet and iodine, after attempted decolorisation with acetone. Gram-negative bacteria fail to retain these stains after the application of acetone. In order to be able to see the organisms they have to be counterstained, usually with basic fuchsin, when they appear pink on microscopy. Although microscopic appearance and Gram-staining reaction of bacteria are the chief means of preliminary identification and classification further studies including cultural, serological and biochemical may be required to complete the classification (Table 2.1).

The currently accepted classification of bacteria is published in *Bergey's Manual of Determinative Bacteriology*. Because this Manual is published infrequently it is inevitable that not all the work is up to date and not all of the recommendations set out in it are accepted by microbiologists, but it is an important publication incorporating international views on classification of microorganisms.

TABLE 2.1   Characteristics used in the identification and classification of bacteria.

Shape
Gram reaction
Ability to grow: in air
                in the absence of air
                in carbon dioxide
                on different media
                at different temperatures
Ability to produce acid from various carbohydrates
Ability to break down various amino-acids
Morphological appearance of colonies
Motility in liquid or semi-solid media
Antigenic characteristics
Enzyme and toxin production
Antibiotic sensitivity
Detailed analysis of the components of the cell wall
Analysis of the DNA composition

The various tests used to identify and classify microorganisms are only performed to the extent required for the particular purpose in hand. For example, clinical specimens often require only limited identification whereas taxonomic studies or epidemiological studies require a much more detailed identification of an organism. Bacteria are usually described by a generic and a species name, for example *Streptococcus* (genus) *mutans* (species).

The term strain is applied to the progeny of one bacterium dividing asexually in primary culture, subculture or in the natural habitat. Species are closely related to each other in fundamental activities but may differ in several minor ways. The genus is a broader group of related species, and is a subdivision of the Family and Order.

Table 2.2. provides a simple classification of the bacteria referred to in this book. The reader is directed to the more detailed texts on microbial taxonomy and classification given at the end of the chapter.

Classification of viruses

Viruses are small intracellular parasites (Chap. 4) that are classified on the basis of (1) shape and structure as viewed in an electronmicroscope; (2) nucleic acid content; (3) chemical composition of the proteins; (4) serological tests; (5) cultural appearances after inoculation of eggs or tissue culture cell lines; and (6) susceptibility to physical and chemical agents. Whereas electronmicroscopic, cultural and serological tests are usually suitable for identification of viruses the more detailed classification of viruses and the understanding of the relationship between different groups of viruses fall within the provinces of molecular biology, biochemistry and genetics. A simple classification of viruses is given in Table 2.3.

Classification of fungi

Fungi are eukaryotic cells of the Kingdom Eumycetae and are of considerable economic and medical importance. These include: (1) mushrooms; (2) brewers' and bakers' yeasts; (3) a number of species that produce antibiotics; and (4) moulds. Some are pathogenic to man and animals. The classification of fungi is complex and is based on the characteristics of the sexually-reproductive or perfect state. Unfortunately this state has not been described in several important fungi and these are grouped together in the Fungi imperfecti. A simple division of fungi into groups that bear more relation to their morphology and pathogenic similarities than to taxonomic principles is as follows:

Yeasts. Classified among the imperfect fungi, these are unicellular fungi that reproduce by budding. Some genera (for example *Candida*) have an alternative form in which long filaments are produced which join end-to-end to form a 'pseudomycelium'. Representative genera: *Candida, Torulopsis, Cryptococcus, Paracoccidioides.*

Filamentous fungi. These organisms produce an interlacing network of filaments or hyphae that constitute the mycelium. Aerial spore-bearing bodies (conidia) are seen and the structure of these is important in the classification of the organism. Most organisms in this group belong to the Class *Ascomycetes*, subdivided in the following way:

	Class Ascomycetes		
Order	*Onygenales*	Order	*Eurotiales*
Represen-	*Trichophyton*	Represen-	*Aspergillus*
tative	*Microsporum*	tative	*Penicillium*
genera	*Histoplasma*	genera	

TABLE 2.2   The classification of bacteria.

Kingdom   Prokaryotae
Division   Bacteria

Genus	Representative species

GRAM-POSITIVE BACTERIA

(1) AEROBIC AND FACULTATIVELY ANAEROBIC COCCI
  (a) *Staphylococcus*   aureus
                          albus
  (b) *Micrococcus*   mucilagenous
  (c) *Streptococcus*   beta haemolytic streptococci
                        mutans ⎤
                        mitior (mitis) ⎥
                        sanguis ⎬ viridans
                        salivarius ⎥ streptococci
                        milleri ⎦
                        faecalis (enterococcus)
                        pneumoniae (pneumococcus)

(2) ANAEROBIC COCCI

(3) AEROBIC AND FACULTATIVELY ANAEROBIC
    SPORE-FORMING RODS
  Bacillus   anthracis

(4) ANAEROBIC SPORE-FORMING RODS
  Clostridium   perfringens (welchii)
                  tetani
                  botulinum

(5) NON-SPORE-FORMING RODS
  (a) *Lactobacillus*   casei
                        acidophilus
  (b) *Corynebacterium*   diphtheriae
  (c) *Propioni-*   acnes
      bacterium   parvum
  (d) *Listeria*   monocytogenes
  (e) *Eubacterium*   saburreum
                      alactolyticum

(6) BRANCHING AND NON-BRANCHING FILAMENTS
  (a) *Actinomyces*   israelii
                      odontolyticus
                      viscosus/naeslundii
  (b) *Arachnia*   propionica
  (c) *Rothia*   dentocariosa
  (d) *Bifidobacterium*   bifidum
                          dentium
  (e) *Bacterionema*   matruchotti

(7) ACID-FAST BACILLI
  Mycobacterium   tuberculosis
                    bovis
                    leprae
                    ulcerans

GRAM-NEGATIVE BACTERIA

(1) AEROBIC AND FACULTATIVELY ANAEROBIC COCCI
  (a) *Neisseria*   gonorrhoeae (gonococcus)
                    meningitidis (meningococcus)
                    pharyngis (N. flava, N. sicca)
  (b) *Branhamella*   catarrhalis

Kingdom   Prokaryotae
Division   Bacteria

Genus	Representative species

(2) ANAEROBIC COCCI
  Veillonella   alkalescens
                  parvula

(3) AEROBIC RODS
  (a) *Pseudomonas*   aeruginosa
  (b) *Bordetella*   pertussis ⎤
  (c) *Brucella*   abortus ⎬ coccobacilli
  (d) *Legionella*   pneumophila ⎦

(4) FACULTATIVELY ANAEROBIC RODS
  (a) *Escherichia*   coli ⎤
  (b) *Klebsiella*   aerogenes ⎥
                     pneumoniae ⎥
  (c) *Proteus*   mirabilis ⎥
                  vulgaris ⎬ the
  (d) *Salmonella*   typhi ⎥ enterobacteria
                     paratyphi ⎥
                     typhimurium ⎥
                     enteritidis ⎥
  (e) *Shigella*   dysenteriae ⎥
                   sonnei ⎦
  (f) *Yersinia*   enterocolitica ⎤ cocco-
  (g) *Pasteurella*   multocida ⎬ bacilli
  (h) *Actinobacillus*   actinomycetemcomitans ⎦
  (i) *Haemophilus*   influenzae
                      segnis
  (j) *Eikenella*   corrodens
  (k) *Capnocytophaga*   ochracea ⎤
                         sputigena ⎬ CO_2 dependent
                         gingivalis ⎦

(5) MOTILE CURVED RODS
  (a) *Vibrio*   cholerae (facultatively anaerobic)
  (b) *Campylobacter*   sputorum ⎤ microaerophilic
                        jejuni ⎦
  (c) *Wolinella*   recta ⎤
                    succinogenes ⎬ anaerobic
  (d) *Selenomonas*   sputigena (anaerobic)

(6) ANAEROBIC RODS AND FILAMENTS
  (a) *Bacteroides*   melaninogenicus ⎤
                      oralis/ruminicola ⎥ saccharolytic
                      fragilis ⎥
                      thetaiotaomicron ⎦
                      asaccharolyticus
                      gingivalis ⎤ saccharolytic
                      ureolyticus ⎦
  (b) *Fusobacterium*   nucleatum
  (c) *Leptotrichia*   buccalis

(7) SPIRAL FORMS
  Spirochaetes
  (a) *Treponema*   pallidum
                    vincenti
                    buccale
                    macrodentium
  (b) *Borrelia*   recurrentis
  (c) *Leptospira*   icterohaemorrhagiae
                     canicola

TABLE 2.3   Simple classification of viruses.

Type of nucleic acid: DNA

Capsid symmetry	Cubic				Complex
Presence of envelope	+	−			...
Sensitivity to ether	S	R			R
Number of capsomeres	162	32	72	252	...
Family	Herpesviridae	Parvoviridae	Papovaviridae	Adenoviridae	Poxviridae
Genus	Herpes simplex virus Cytomegalovirus Epstein–Barr virus	Parvovirus	Wart virus	Adenovirus	Variola (smallpox virus)

Type of nucleic acid: RNA

Capsid symmetry	Cubic			Helical		
Presence of envelope	+	−		+		
Sensitivity to ether	S	R		S		
Number of capsomeres	32	32		...		
Family	Togaviridae	Reoviridae	Picorna-viridae	Rhabdo-viridae	Paramyxo-viridae	Orthomyxo-viridae
Genus	Rubella	Reovirus	(1) Enterovirus Poliovirus Coxsackie virus Echo virus (2) Rhinovirus	Rabies virus	Parainfluenza virus Mumps virus Measles virus	Influenza virus

---

S = Sensitive;   R = Resistant;   . . . not recorded

Classification of microorganisms intermediate between bacteria and viruses

Three small groups of important prokaryotic microorganisms are difficult to place in either the bacterial or viral classification. They are the orders *Mycoplasmatales, Rickettsiales* and *Chlamydiales.*

Mycoplasmatales: These organisms have no true bacterial cell wall but in other respects resemble bacteria. They can be cultured on artificial media and the principal genus, *Mycoplasma* includes several species found in the mouth, for example *Mycoplasma orale, Mycoplasma buccale* and *Mycoplasma salivarium.*

Rickettsiales: These microorganisms are obligate intracellular parasites and often appear as rod-like bodies. They have a bacterial type of cell wall and possess DNA, RNA and enzymes capable of cleaving high-energy-yielding bonds. Thus they differ significantly from viruses. Two principal genera are known, *Coxiella* and *Rickettsia.*

Chlamydiales: There is one genus, *Chlamydia;* the two species are *Chlamydia trachomatis* and *Chlamydia psittaci,* Gram-negative obligate intracellular parasites that replicate within the host cell. They possess DNA and RNA but, like viruses, are not capable of cleaving high-energy-yielding bonds.

FURTHER READING

Bergey's Manual of Determinative Bacteriology (1974) 8th Edition. Baltimore: Williams and Wilkins.

Duguid J.P., Marmion B.P. & Swain R.H.A., eds (1978) *Mackie and McCartney Medical Microbiology*, 13th Edition. Edinburgh: Churchill Livingstone.

Lenette E.H., Balows A., Hausler, W.J. & Truant J.P. (1980). *Manual of Clinical Microbiology*, 3rd Edition. Washington: American Society for Microbiology.

Milne L.J.R. (1980) Mycology. In *A Companion to Medical Studies*, Vol. 2, 2nd Edition. Chapter 23, eds Passmore R. & Robson J.S. Oxford: Blackwell Scientific Publications.

Timbury Morag C. (1978) *Notes on Medical Virology*, 6th Edition. Edinburgh: Churchill Livingstone.

CHAPTER 3

Morphology and Physiology of Bacteria and Fungi

BACTERIA

The bacterial cell (Fig. 3.1)

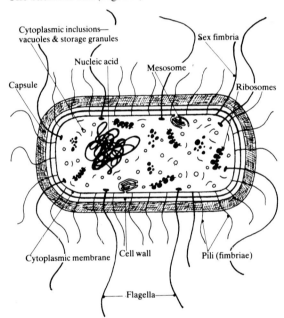

FIG. 3.1. A composite bacterial cell.

The bacterial cell is bound by a rigid cell wall that is porous and permeable. This cell wall is composed of molecules of N-acetylglucosamine and N-acetyl-muramic acid linked alternately in chains. Peptide side chains are attached to the N-acetylmuramic acid molecules and these in turn are cross-linked by other peptides giving a rigid structure that possesses some elasticity.

This forms the basic structure of the cell wall. Supplementing the basic structure are special struc-tures such as teichoic acids, polysaccharides and polypeptides or proteins, that account for 20 per cent of the cell wall weight in *Staphylococcus aureus* but 80 per cent in Gram-negative organisms such as *Escherichia*. There are considerable species differ-ences in the composition of the supplementary struc-ture of the cell wall (Fig. 3.2).

The cell wall is sometimes surrounded by a capsule, as in *Streptococcus pneumoniae* and *Klebsiella*,

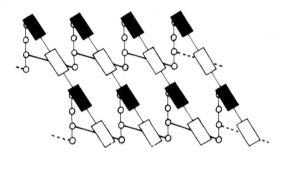

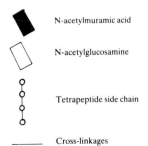

N-acetylmuramic acid

N-acetylglucosamine

Tetrapeptide side chain

Cross-linkages

FIG. 3.2. The peptidoglycan polymer of bacterial cell walls.

consisting of proteins and polysaccharides. The capsule may have a protective function for the cell preventing phagocytosis in some instances. Possession of a capsule is one of the factors that increases the pathogenicity of an organism. Capsules can act as antigens and this feature is utilised in diagnostic bacteriology.

All the protoplasm inside the cell wall is collectively termed the protoplast. This is bound by the cytoplasmic membrane which is a thin elastic semipermeable structure that permits passively the passage of water and small molecules. Other molecules crossing this barrier are actively transported. The cytoplasmic membrane is composed of phospholipid molecules arranged in a bilayer in which protein molecules are embedded (Fig. 3.3).

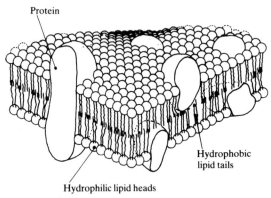

FIG. 3.3. Unit membrane that forms the cytoplasmic membrane of a bacterium.

The bounding layers of Gram-positive cells differ in arrangement from Gram-negative cells, although this was not known to Gram when his staining procedure was proposed. The walls of Gram-positive cells are arranged as described above with the cytoplasmic membrane covered by the cell wall which in turn may be surrounded by a capsule (Fig. 3.4). The arrangement of the Gram-negative cell wall is somewhat different (Fig. 3.5). Here the cytoplasmic membrane again surrounds the cytoplasm and a thin layer of peptidoglycan surrounds the cytoplasmic membrane. There is then a space, the periplasmic space containing lipoprotein and numerous enzymes. This space is bound to the exterior by a second phospholipid-bilayer membrane containing structural proteins and enzymes. Many Gram-negative cells are surrounded by a capsule.

The cytoplasm of bacteria contains numerous ribosomes often arranged on folds of membrane and termed a mesosome. Inclusion bodies and storage granules may also be present in some bacteria. The DNA of the bacterial cells is not confined by a nuclear membrane but consists of a loop of double-stranded nucleic acid tightly coiled up. It divides by simple fission and not by mitosis.

Some bacteria possess flagella or organs of motility. These long filaments consist of contractile proteins and may be single or multiple.

Flagella may be arranged around the cell or located at one or both poles of the bacterium.

Many bacteria possess fimbriae (or pili) that are filamentous appendages surrounding the bacterium, much more numerous than flagella and shorter. These are thought to be organs of adherence and several types have been described. One special long

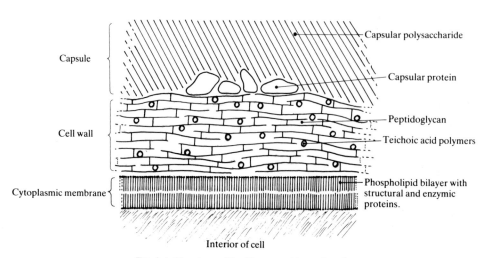

FIG. 3.4. Structure of the Gram-positive cell wall.

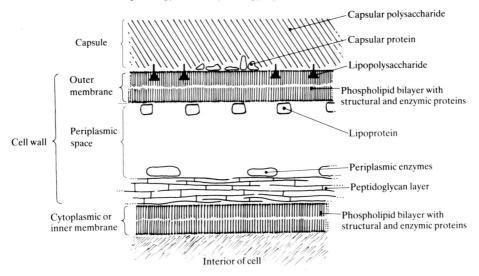

FIG. 3.5. Structure of the Gram-negative cell wall.

fimbria appears to be the organ of sexual conjugation between bacteria.

Spores are resistant forms produced by some bacteria that enable the organism to survive adverse conditions. One spore gives rise to a new vegetative cell when favourable conditions return. Some spores, for example *Clostridium tetani*, can remain dormant for many years. The location of a spore in a vegetative cell is often a helpful morphological feature in identification of the organism, for example the genus *Clostridium*.

Spheroplasts and L-forms

In unfavourable conditions such as nutrient deficient media or in the presence of antibiotics bacteria may grow in a form in which the cell wall is rudimentary or absent. Sometimes these forms are stable and reproduce (L-forms); others revert to normal bacterial morphology on restoration of normal conditions (Spheroplasts). Members of the genus *Bacteroides* isolated from the mouth often appear on initial culture as spheroplasts and revert to their normal Gram-negative cocco-bacillary form on subculture.

Bacterial growth and physiology

All bacteria require carbon, energy and nitrogen sources for growth but they vary greatly in their ability to synthesise compounds. A few bacteria can utilise gaseous nitrogen but most need an ammonium salt and some require pre-formed amino-acids in their environment that can be absorbed when required.

Several organic growth factors and inorganic mineral salts may also be required, a direct parallel with the requirement of man for vitamins and minerals. The synthesis of amino-acids and proteins requires energy which is made available in the form of ATP. ATP is produced from ADP and the energy produced largely from the breakdown of organic compounds. Again bacteria differ widely in their ability to break down organic compounds: this factor is made much use of in bacterial identification tests.

Bacteria may grow in the presence or absence of oxygen (Table 3.1). In fact bacteria are more accurately described as being susceptible to the overall state of oxidation or reduction of their surroundings — the oxidation-reduction potential (Eh). This can be measured in bacterial cultures using a platinum electrode and a standard calomel electrode.

TABLE 3.1   The effect of oxygen on the growth of bacteria.

Degree of oxygenation	Term	Example
Oxygen required for growth	Obligate aerobe	*Pseudomonas aeruginosa*
Only low oxygen concentration preferred (5%)	Microaerophile	*Campylobacter fetus*
Grows in presence or absence of oxygen	Facultative anaerobe	*Escherichia coli*
Only grows in absence of oxygen	Obligate anaerobe	*Bacteroides melanino-genicus*

If an organism obtains its energy by a series of biochemical reactions in which the terminal electron acceptor is oxygen this is termed aerobic respiration. Some organisms are able to respire anaerobically using sulphate or nitrate as the electron acceptor. Most anaerobic metabolism yields energy, however, by the process of fermentation that produces a variety of waste products such as alcohols or organic acids.

In vitro, bacteria multiply rapidly (and they may also do so *in vivo*) under favourable conditions. Multiplication is by binary fission and results in a characteristic growth curve when numbers of bacteria are plotted against time (Fig. 3.6).

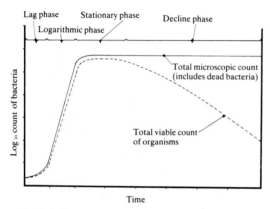

FIG. 3.6. Curve to show the multiplication of bacteria with time.

When a small number of organisms (an inoculum) is placed into fresh growth medium no immediate increase in numbers is observed. This period of adaptation to the new medium is termed the lag phase and it varies with species of organism and the physical conditions. Bacterial multiplication begins and continues at a steady rate so that the logarithm of the number of bacteria plotted against time produces a straight line (Fig. 3.6). This is the logarithmic or log phase. As the nutrients in the medium are exhausted and waste products increase some cells die. However, some continue to divide so that the total count remains much the same. This is known as the stationary phase. After a variable interval more cells die and there is a reduction in the number of viable cells; this is the decline phase. The length of the stationary phase and the steepness of the decline phase are both governed by the culture medium, the physical conditions and the organism involved.

In the body the normal bacterial flora is continuously renewed and attempts have been made to reproduce such a continuous culture system in the laboratory. These culture systems are called chemostats and they have been most helpful in the study of the interaction of organisms. There is considerable potential for further studies on the oral flora with such apparatus. In principle fresh medium is added and older medium removed in such a way that the increase in cells is equilibrated by the loss of cells.

Laboratory culture of bacteria and yeasts

In the laboratory culture of bacteria and yeasts is possible using growth media. These are usually in liquid form (broth media) or solidified with agar, a gelatin-like material derived from seaweed. Liquid and solid media may be dispensed, sterile and ready for use, in test tubes or bottles and solid media are commonly dispensed in sterile flat dishes called Petri dishes or plates that have a closely fitting lid (Fig. 3.7).

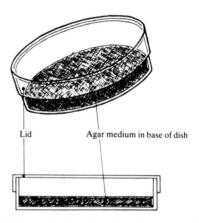

FIG. 3.7. Petri dish for cultivation of bacteria and fungi on solid media.

In the laboratory bacteria are transferred from one culture to fresh medium by means of a sterile loop, usually wire, that picks up a small drop of fluid culture or part of a colony of a bacterium growing on solid medium. The sample is then placed in fresh liquid medium or spread across the surface of solid media usually in such a manner as to yield a well-spread culture. Straight wires, swabs and Pasteur pipettes are also used for inoculating media. It is assumed that one viable bacterium in an inoculum will give rise to one colony after incubation. This is often demonstrated by diluting an inoculum in ten-fold steps and counting the number of colonies that grow from each dilution. A ten-fold decrease in viable counts is observed with increasing dilution.

With mixed cultures it is necessary to spread the inoculum across the surface of the medium in order to obtain separate colonies of each organism in the mixture. The individual colonies are then more easily picked from the plate and can be grown subsequently in pure subculture (Fig. 3.8).

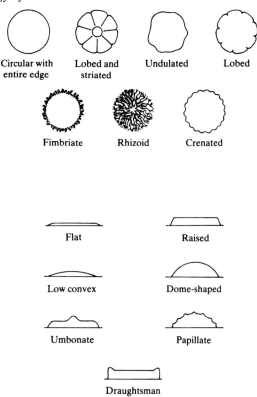

FIG. 3.9. The shapes of bacterial colonies.

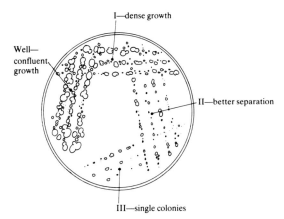

FIG. 3.8. Plating out of a specimen on to agar. Part of the specimen is used to inoculate a well. Subsequent series of strokes I, II, & III are made with flaming of the loop between changes of direction to produce single colonies that can be more easily subcultured.

Bacterial colonies

Bacteria grown on solid media give rise to colonies which may be of assistance in the identification of the organism. Colonies are usually circular, convex and have an entire edge. The variety of morphological appearances of bacterial colonies is shown in Fig. 3.9. Colour may vary enormously depending on both medium and intrinsic properties of the organism. In liquid cultures of bacteria an even turbidity is usually seen but occasionally organisms grow in clumps or microcolonies and the medium appears granular.

Products from the bacterial colony may have an effect on the medium, such as the haemolysis seen when streptococci are grown on blood agar. This may be complete (β) or incomplete resulting in a narrow zone of green coloration around the colony (α). Protein digesting or coagulating enzymes, lipases, DNAses and other enzyme products may be demonstrated by culturing certain bacteria on special media. The enzyme then produces a recognisable effect in the medium. Some bacteria such as *Bacteroides melaninogenicus* produce pigmented colonies, and some such as *Pseudomonas aeruginosa* produce pigment in the medium. Other coloured colonies may be the result of an indicator changing colour in the medium as a result of bacterial fermentation of certain sugars; the pink colonies of *Escherichia coli* on MacConkey's medium exemplify this.

Media

Growth media may be general in that they support the growth of a wide range of bacteria and/or fungi and these often contain nonspecific extracts or digests of meat or other protein. Sometimes simple or complex defined media are used in which the chemical nature of all the constituents is known. Media can be supplemented to allow them to be used to select out a few microorganisms from a mixed culture by inhibiting the growth of others. These selective media often contain antibiotics, bile or other inhibitory substances. Sometimes liquid media are supplemented with growth factors for one organism and inhibitory factors for others. This allows small numbers of one organism to multiply sufficiently to be detected. Such media are termed enrichment media.

Many substances, for example carbohydrates, are included in media for the purpose of carrying out identification tests on microorganisms. Growth or failure to grow in these media and effects on the media, such as carbohydrate fermentation, form the basis of many laboratory tests in microbiology that help identify and characterise microorganisms.

Physical conditions

It is necessary to ensure that the physical conditions for growth of microorganisms in the laboratory are appropriate and many such factors have been found to affect their culture. The temperature at which the bacteria are growing is most important. Whereas most human pathogens have optimum growth temperatures of around 37°C, organisms from the environment may have optimum temperatures lower or higher than this. In clinical microbiology laboratories fungi, including yeasts, are generally grown at 22–28°C whereas most bacterial cultures are performed at 37°C. The pH of the medium must be considered and although clinical isolates will usually grow close to pH 7 tolerance of lower pH levels may be an important aspect of the pathogenicity of the organism *in vivo* and many facilitate isolation and identification *in vitro*. The oxidation-reduction potential (Eh) of the incubation atmosphere is crucial to the culture of all but facultative organisms. Anaerobic organisms are usually placed in an anaerobic jar prior to incubation. This apparatus (Fig. 3.10) can be evacuated after closing and re-filled with an oxygen-free gas mixture containing 90 per cent H_2 and 10 per cent CO_2 or 80 per cent N_2, 10

per cent H_2 and 10 per cent CO_2. The catalyst pellets of alumina coated with palladium are contained in a sachet in the lid of the jar and combine residual oxygen with hydrogen to produce water. Chemical generation of hydrogen and carbon dioxide in a jar may be achieved with a 'Gas-Pak' or similar system. The jar is placed in an incubator to maintain the correct temperature. Recent developments in the technology of working with anaerobic bacteria have included cabinets that allow all handling of these microorganisms and their incubation to be carried out in an oxygen-free atmosphere. Some microorganisms grow better in the presence of an increased carbon-dioxide concentration (5–10%) and the incorporation of this may enhance growth markedly. Such organisms may be strict anaerobes (*Bacteroides* spp) or facultative anaerobes (*Streptococcus pygogenes*) or they may, rarely, have an absolute requirement for CO_2 such as the oral organism *Capnocytophaga ochracea*.

It is important to provide appropriate nutrients for the growth of any particular microorganism but in mixed culture competition from other organisms may well inhibit growth of the desired species. In older cultures and frequently in mixed cultures where one organism multiplies rapidly exhaustion of growth substances and accumulation of waste products in the medium may drastically affect further growth.

All microorganisms are susceptible to desiccation and growth media and incubation atmosphere should be kept moist to avoid loss of viability of the culture. Many microorganisms are susceptible to light, especially ultra-violet radiation.

Disruption of a bacterial culture by ultrasonic vibration reduces its viability and is sometimes used in the laboratory. The use of ultrasonic scalers in the mouth to remove calculus and dental plaque may therefore have a bactericidal effect as well as one of mechanical removal of the deposits. Ultrasonic vibration is used to disrupt plaque samples for bacteriological examination but this is usually carried out in such a way as to keep the loss of viability to a minimum.

FUNGI

Fungi are eukaryotes, are more complex than bacteria and exhibit quite varied morphology. Several fungi even possess two basic forms (dimorphism).

Yeasts

Yeasts are unicellular with oval or spherical cells 2–5 μm in diameter and stain positively by Gram's

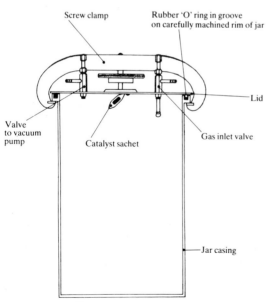

Screw clamp   Rubber 'O' ring in groove on carefully machined rim of jar

Valve to vacuum pump

Catalyst sachet

Gas inlet valve

Lid

Jar casing

FIG. 3.10. An anaerobic jar.

method. They are usually seen with lateral projections or buds which represent daughter cells that increase in size until they split off from the parent cell. Yeasts of the genus *Candida*, one of the most important fungi in the mouth, may also produce a pseudomycelial form comprising a network of interlacing filaments. This differs from true mycelium in having numerous cross-walls. *Candida albicans* is also characterised by its ability to produce a small projection of protoplasm from the yeast cell, the germ tube, when incubated in the presence of serum. This species may also produce dormant forms resembling bacterial spores at the end of a filament — chlamydospores (Fig. 3.11).

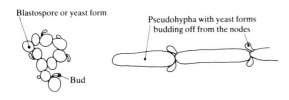

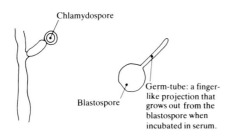

FIG. 3.11. The forms of *Candida albicans*.

Filamentous fungi

These forms grow as an interlacing network (mycelium) of filaments (hyphae). An aerial fruiting body containing spores is often seen and on germination of a spore the hollow-tubed hypha grows out. Fungi of the genus *Histoplasma* grow as filamentous fungi in nature but may be pathogenic for man when they are found in a yeast-like form. Environmental factors such as Eh and temperature are important in determining the nature of the form found. The structure of the spore-bearing aerial forms are especially important in identification of the fungi that produce them (for example, *Aspergillus, Penicillium, Trichophyton, Microsporum).*

Cytology

The cell walls of fungi contain chitin, a polymer of N-acetylglucosamine, which is also found in the exoskeleton of insects. As they are eukaryotes the nucleus is well differentiated with a nuclear membrane and in many respects they resemble lower plants.

Growth of fungi

Fungi are facultative anaerobes that grow slowly compared with bacteria. It is not possible to generalise about fungi as they include such a wide range of organisms. Most will, however, grow on relatively simple media and although the range of optimal temperatures is wide most will grow in the range 20–28°C. A few are inhibited by incubation at 37°C and most by temperatures above 45°C. Fungi need a source of carbohydrate such as sucrose, malt or starch. They are able to tolerate well the low pH that develops when these carbohydrates are broken down. A general purpose fungal growth medium such as Sabouraud's or malt extract medium is used to inhibit the growth of bacteria. Fungi do not have a bacterial type of cell wall and thus are not susceptible to antibacterial drugs.

Although fungi grow slowly the stationary phase, once reached, may last for a long time and the decline phase proceeds slowly. It is possible to keep a refrigerated culture of a yeast for a year and still successfully subculture from it.

Yeasts grow as circular white or cream colonies on solid media; the consistency of the colony is characteristically like cream cheese. Better morphological differentiation of yeasts is seen on malt agar rather than on Sabouraud's. The filamentous fungi (moulds and the dermatophytes) are characterised by their production of aerial sporing bodies. Some also produce pigmentation of the colony, for example the red colour of *Trichophyton rubrum*. The colonies tend to be large and spreading with a wrinkled appearance that is often covered by a velvety sheen.

FURTHER READING

Davis B.D., Dulbecco R., Eisen H.N. & Ginsberg H.S. eds (1980) *Microbiology*, 3rd Edition. New York: Harper and Row.
Duguid J.P., Marmion B.P. and Swain R.H.A. eds (1978) *Mackie and McCartney Medical Microbiology*, 13th Edition. Edinburgh: Churchill Livingstone.

CHAPTER 4

Viruses

Structure of viruses

Viruses are difficult to describe but the following definition of Luria is helpful. 'Viruses are entities whose genomes are elements of nucleic acid that replicate inside living cells using the cellular synthetic machinery and causing the synthesis of specialised elements that can transfer the viral genome to other cells'.

Viruses therefore differ significantly from bacteria in structure in that they have no rigid cell wall, no muramic acid in the outer coverings and no ribosomes. They have no mitochondria and do not possess enzymes capable of forming high energy bonds ($ADP + P \rightarrow ATP$). Although the structure of viruses is diverse some common features are to be found. The complete infective particle is termed the virion and its nucleic acid core is the genome. All viruses have an outer shell of protein, the capsid, composed of aggregations of polypeptide capsomeres and some have an outer envelope derived from host cell membrane which may contain small amounts of lipid and sometimes carbohydrate. Fig. 4.1 demonstrates the morphology of certain viruses.

Projecting from the nucleocapsid there are polypeptide units such as haemagglutinins that give the virus a haemagglutinating activity, and neuraminidase subunits that play a part in the attachment of the virus to host cells. These polypeptide units project through any envelope that may be present. The protein forming the capsid is often antigenic and may stimulate the host response to viral infection.

The nucleic acid itself may be a double or a single strand or may be circular. Most DNA viruses have a double-stranded nucleic acid, whereas it is single-stranded in most RNA viruses. This nucleic acid is symmetrically arranged within the nucleocapsid, often helically.

Pox virus
Example: Molluscum
   contagiosum
   virus

Paramyxovirus
Example: Mumps virus

Herpes virus

Examples:
Herpes simplex virus
Varicella-zoster virus
Epstein-Barr virus

Orthomyxovirus
Example: Influenza virus

Coronavirus
Example: Rhinovirus

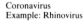
Adenovirus

Bacteriophage

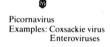
Picornavirus
Examples: Coxsackie virus
     Enteroviruses

FIG. 4.1. Morphology of viruses.

Physical properties of viruses

Viruses are highly susceptible to killing during any period they are outside their animal host, although some viruses such as *Variola* (causative agent of smallpox) polio virus and hepatitis virus are relatively hardy. Most viruses are killed by temperatures in excess of 50°C but hepatitis virus is an exception. They are usually susceptible to desiccation but resist freezing; indeed freezing is commonly used to preserve viruses.

Those viruses possessing lipid in the envelope, for example mumps virus and herpes virus are susceptible to ether which destroys the envelope. Others, for example adenovirus that do not have a lipid covering are resistant to ether. Viruses are also susceptible to ultraviolet light.

Growth and replication of viruses

Viruses are perhaps the most extreme examples of a parasitic mode of life in that they need to utilise the host cell chemistry in order to reproduce. The direction to the host cell to produce virus rather than host material comes from the successful take-over of cell control by virus messenger RNA.

A virus first recognises specific receptors on the host cell membrane and becomes attached (adsorption), then it passes through the cell membrane into the cytoplasm of the host cell where the envelope and outer protein layer of the virus are stripped off revealing the nucleic acid. For a DNA virus, viral m-RNA is produced using the viral nucleic acid as a template; this m-RNA then governs the production of proteins by ribosomes of the host cell. At first enzymes are produced that are required to synthesise more viral DNA. Later the viral structural proteins are produced and these are coded for by the progeny DNA molecules. Assembly of new viral particles now occurs and then the virus particles pass through the host cell, sometimes acquiring an envelope as they are released.

In RNA viruses the nucleic acid of the infective virus particle may act as m-RNA (positive-strand RNA viruses, for example poliovirus). Alternatively the virus may contain RNA polymerase which transcribes m-RNA of the nucleic acid templates of the infecting particle (negative-strand RNA viruses, for example, mumps or influenza viruses). This m-RNA then governs the production of progeny RNA molecules and structural proteins. Virus particles are then assembled and released, often acquiring an envelope.

Culture of viruses

Viruses can only reproduce inside living cells and therefore media for their culture have itself to be viable, unlike the culture media required for bacteria and fungi which are inanimate. Viruses have been grown by inoculating laboratory animals, although this is done much less frequently today. Inoculation of fertile hens' eggs with virus particles was extensively practised and some grow well in this medium. The advent of tissue culture, however, provided a great improvement in media available for the culture of viruses. Cells for tissue culture may be detached from pieces of tissue by the action of trypsin

and then allowed to settle on the inside of a glass test-tube. The cells are maintained in a viable state by a nutrient tissue-culture fluid containing carbohydrate, proteins, serum and buffer. Antibiotics are also included in order to prevent accidental bacterial contamination and to kill off any bacteria that may be in the sample intended for virus detection. Some tissue cultures can be sustained for much longer periods than the primary cell culture described above. These continuous cell lines are derived from malignant cells and divide rapidly; they can be subcultured by removing some cells and passing them into fresh tissue culture medium. The cells will divide and settle to form a cell layer (monolayer). Semi-continuous cell lines are derived from normal tissue with a potent, natural, capacity to divide, such as embryonic fibroblasts. These can often be passaged for quite long periods.

After receiving the specimen the tubes containing the cell monolayers are inoculated and examined after a few days for the signs of virus multiplication.

Effect of viruses on cells: cytopathic effect

Viruses may kill cells and be released, may remain dormant within a cell, or may alter a cell without killing it. The effect of viral infection on a cell monolayer is termed the cytopathic effect (CPE). When examined by low-power microscopy the CPE of many viruses is often fairly typical and is an important clue to the identity of the type of virus growing (Figs. 4.2, 4.3). Cells of normal cell lines form a continuous sheet but after viral infection the cells become rounded, often swollen and usually drop off, leaving void spaces in the cell sheet. Sometimes cells coalesce to form syncytia.

Identification of viruses

Confirmation of the identity of the virus is often obtained by observing the haemadsorbing ability of infected cells to which added erythrocytes will adhere. The cells may be used in a neutralisation test in which two fresh parallel tubes are inoculated from the one showing a CPE. One of the pair has antibody to the suspected virus added. The monolayer with no antibody present should produce a CPE in the normal way whereas neutralising antibody will protect the other cell monolayer from infection by the virus, thus confirming its identity.

Neutralisation test

Virus + antiserum   culture → no CPE
Virus   culture → CPE

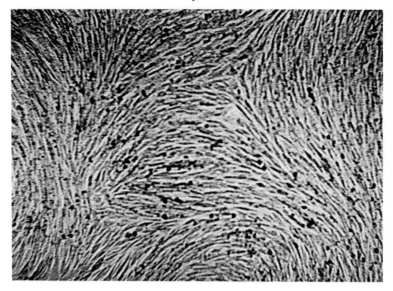

FIG.4.2. Uninfected fibroblast tissue culture. From Grist N.R. *et al* (1979) *Diagnostic Methods in Clinical Virology*, 3rd Edition. Oxford, Blackwell Scientific Publications.

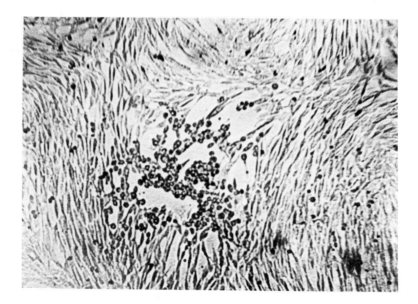

FIG. 4.3. Cytopathic effect (CPE) produced by Herpes simplex type 1 in a fibroblast tissue culture. From Grist N.R. *et al* (1979) *Diagnostic Methods in Clinical Virology*, 3rd Edition. Oxford, Blackwell Scientific Publications.

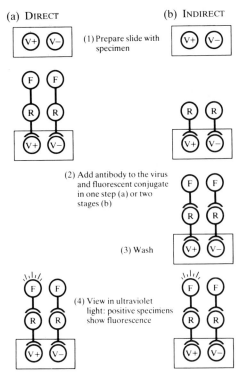

(a) DIRECT (b) INDIRECT

(1) Prepare slide with specimen

(2) Add antibody to the virus and fluorescent conjugate in one step (a) or two stages (b)

(3) Wash

(4) View in ultraviolet light: positive specimens show fluorescence

FIG. 4.4. Diagrammatic representation of the immunofluorescence test for the detection of viruses. V + = virus present; V − = virus absent; R = antibody to the virus raised in a rabbit; F = fluorescent conjugate.

Fluorescence

Fresh specimens or a cell monolayer may be treated with one of a range of specific antibodies to viruses. After washing only antibody directed against the infecting virus will remain. The slide is then treated with fluorescent-labelled antibody to gammaglobulin. This complex of virus-antibody-fluorescent-labelled antibody to gammaglobulin fluoresces when viewed down a microscope equipped with an ultraviolet light source. This has been a useful way of speeding up the identification of viruses (Fig. 4.4).

Electronmicroscopy

In the early stages of suspected virus infections a specimen can be collected and submitted for electronmicroscopic examination (Fig. 4.5). Although this offers a very quick way to identify the likely viral cause there are problems in collecting adequate specimens and transporting them rapidly to the electronmicroscope. Negative results should never be relied upon without cultural or serological tests but a positive result can be especially helpful particularly since it is given quickly, for example in rotavirus infection. It must be remembered that some specimens contain viruses that are not causing any symptoms, and therefore caution is required in interpretation of results.

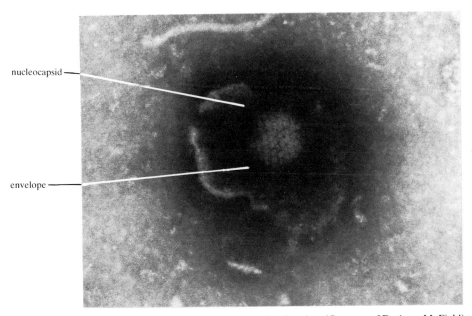

nucleocapsid

envelope

FIG. 4.5. Electronmicrograph of Herpes simplex virus (Courtesy of Dr Anne M. Field).

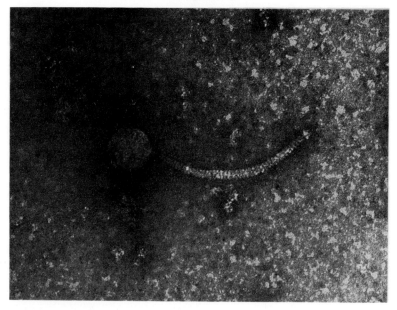

FIG. 4.6. Electronmicrograph of bacteriophage (Courtesy of Dr Anne M. Field).

Serology

One of the most important ways of detecting a viral infection is the detection of antibodies to the virus in the patient's serum. (Chap. 10).

Bacteriophage

Bacteriophages are viruses that parasitise bacteria (Fig. 4.6). There are many different types and they may contain RNA or DNA. The head structure contains the coiled double strand of DNA and there is a central contractile portion from which the long tail-portion stems. Phages adhere to the bacterial cell and then inject their DNA into the bacterium by contraction of the central portion. They are of importance in the study of bacterial genetics and biochemistry and are also used as an epidemiological tool where the susceptibility of bacterial isolates of the same species to a range of phages can be compared in order to determine if the bacteria are of the same strain. This is used in typing *Salmonella* spp, *Staphylococcus aureus* and other bacteria.

FURTHER READING

Luria, S.E., Darnell J.E., Baltimore D. & Campbell A. (1978) *General Virology*, 3rd Edition. New York: John Wiley.

McLean D.M. (1980) *Virology in Health Care*. Baltimore: Williams and Wilkins.

Timbury M.C. (1978) *Notes on Medical Virology*, 6th Edition. Edinburgh: Churchill Livingstone.

CHAPTER 5

Mycoplasmas, Rickettsiae and Chlamydiae

These organisms are intermediate between bacteria and viruses and a comparison of their properties is given in Table 5.1.

Mycoplasmas

These are the smallest prokaryotes capable of growing in cell-free medium. The mycoplasma cell does not possess a rigid cell wall but is bound by a plasma membrane which contains much lipid and sterols. These cells are highly pleomorphic, a factor that depends on the medium. The nuclear material is collected into strands but is not bound by a nuclear membrane. The cytoplasm contains many ribosomes but no lipoprotein membrane structures. Some mycoplasmas are able to break down amino acids and fatty acids whereas others can break down carbohydrates.

Laboratory growth and detection. They are grown aerobically usually in sloppy-agar cultures containing serum and yeast extract in a rich protein base. When grown on such plates the colonies produce a characteristic 'fried-egg' appearance with a central partially-submerged ball surrounded by an outer rim on the agar surface. Mycoplasmas also grow well in tissue culture; indeed they are often an irritating source of contamination of tissue cultures. Since they do not possess a bacterial type of cell wall mycoplasmas are not sensitive to the antibiotics that prevent cell-wall formation such as penicillin but they are susceptible to tetracyclines and erythromycin. Infection with mycoplasmas is usually detected serologically.

Rickettsiae

These microorganisms are obligate intracellular parasites but in other ways resemble bacteria. Organisms of the genus *Rickettsia* are small pleomorphic rods and are Gram negative. *Coxiella*, on the other hand, stains Gram positive although these two genera are still thought to be related, and are included in the same family (Rickettsiaceae).

The structure of the rickettsial cell closely resembles that of other Gram-negative bacteria, with a multi-layered outer membrane (some rickettsiae are capsulate), cytoplasm containing ribosomes and

TABLE 5.1.

	Bacteria	Mycoplasmas	Rickettsiae	Chlamydiae	Viruses
Capable of free growth	+	+	−	−	−
DNA and RNA present	+	+	+	+	−
Enzymes capable of cleaving high energy bonds	+	+	+	−	−
Muramic acid in cell wall	+	+	+	+	−
Rigid cell wall	+	−	+	Variable	Variable
Susceptible to penicillin	+	−	−	−	−
Susceptible to tetracycline	+	+	+	+	−
Reproduce essentially by binary fission	+	+	+	+	−

nuclear material not bound by a separate nuclear membrane. The chemical composition of the cell wall also resembles that of Gram-negative cell walls and contains n-acetylmuramic acid, n-acetylglucosamine and diaminopimelic acid. Like bacteria the rickettsiae multiply by binary fission. They possess enzymes for the generation of ATP and can synthesise lipid and protein but their intracellular existence allows for a ready supply of pre-formed compounds. *Coxiella burneti* is a rather more robust organism in being quite resistant to heat up to 60°C, drying, and phenolic disinfectants, and can remain viable for long periods outside the body.

Laboratory growth and detection: Rickettsiae cause a variety of diseases such as typhus, a group of spotted fevers and other fevers. *Coxiella burneti* causes Q-fever. All these organisms present a potential danger to laboratory workers and as a consequence their growth and isolation is restricted to specialised laboratories where containment facilities are available. Early workers propagated these microorganisms in experimental animals or in the yolk sac of fertile hens' eggs, a hazardous procedure that has now been replaced by the use of cell culture. Growth is rather slow but when infection is suspected a suspension can be injected into two animals, one protected with specific antiserum and the other not. The organism will usually kill the unprotected animal rapidly, whereas the other will survive.

Chlamydiae. These prokaryotes are also highly specialised for an intracellular parasitic existence. Like rickettsiae they are small Gram-negative organisms that reproduce by binary fission. The cell walls are similar in structure to Gram-negative bacteria and the cells contain both DNA and RNA. During the life cycle of these organisms two morphological forms are known to exist. Small elementary bodies are the infectious agents that invade a new host cell whereupon there is an increase in RNA synthesis. The elementary body enlarges to about three or four times its size, forming a less-densely stained reticulate body, the form of the organism which divides by binary fission.

Clinical specimens and cell cultures infected with chlamydiae show inclusion bodies which stain with Giemsa's stain or iodine (for *Chlamydia trachomatis*). These inclusion bodies consist of reticulate and elementary bodies with a glycogen matrix in *Chlamydia trachomatis*. Glycogen is not found in *Chlamydia psittaci*.

Laboratory growth and detection. Diagnosis of chlamydial infection may be made:

(1) serologically (complement fixation test).

(2) by staining or fluorescent-antibody staining of direct smears from the lesion.

(3) by growth in tissue culture.

Chlamydia trachomatis is successfully grown in tissue culture (McCoy cells) when inclusion bodies should be seen which can be stained with iodine, Giemsa or with an immunofluorescent stain. Animal inoculation is also possible as is growth of the agent in the yolk sac of fertile hens' eggs. These latter procedures present considerable hazard to laboratory staff working with *Chlamydia psittaci*.

FURTHER READING

Cruickshank R., Duguid J.P., Marmion B.P. & Swain R.H.A. (1975) *Medical Microbiology* Vol. II, 12th Edition. Edinburgh: Churchill Livingstone.

Lenette E.H., Balows E., Hausler W.J. & Truant J.P. (1980) *Manual of Clinical Microbiology,* 3rd Edition Washington: The American Society for Microbiology.

Taylor-Robinson D. & Thomas B.J. (1980) The role of *Chlamydia trachomatis* in genital tract and associated diseases. *Journal of Clinical Pathology,* **33,** 205–33.

Timbury M.C. (1978) *Notes on Medical Virology* 6th Edition Edinburgh: Churchill Livingstone.

CHAPTER 6

Sources and Spread of Infections

THE SOURCE OF INFECTIONS

The source of an infection refers to the habitat or growth area in the human or animal. Reservoir and vehicle refer to objects that are contaminated or colonised by microorganisms; for example fingers may be the vehicle for staphylococci derived from a reservoir in the anterior nares.

Infections may be endogenous (autogenous) or exogenous.

Many areas of the body have a normal commensal flora characteristic of the particular area, which has many functions including the provision of a barrier to infection in the individual. Occasionally organisms of the normal flora can cause infection; for example, two species of the viridans streptococci, *Streptococcus sanguis* and *mitior,* may produce infection in previously damaged heart valves when they enter the bloodstream from the mouth following dental extraction. Dental caries is also an endogenous infection. Other examples of endogenous infections include osteomyelitis in which *Staphylococcus aureus* may have been derived from a septic lesion in the skin, and infection of burns by beta-haemolytic streptococci from the patient's own upper respiratory tract. There are two common features in endogenous infections. Firstly they are frequently a manifestation of lowered tissue resistance or tissue damage; and secondly, problems of endogenous infections are generally confined to the patient, in that they do not normally constitute high cross-infection risks.

Exogenous infections are derived from man, animals or the soil. Man is the most common source of exogenous infection, either when the patient is suffering from clinical infection or when the person is a carrier of infection. In whooping cough, smallpox and influenza where the carrier state is thought not to exist, or at least to be of minimal importance in the transmission of infection, the clinical case is the source and such patients represent a major danger in the spread of these infections. Virus infections are almost always exogenous.

Infections are commonly contracted from carriers and various types of these are described, such as healthy, convalescent and chronic. Healthy carriers harbour organisms in their tissues without showing any signs of clinical infection and because of this they constitute a particularly dangerous form of carrier. Streptococcal sore throat, various types of pneumonia and meningococcal meningitis can be contracted in this way as can intestinal infections such as bacillary dysentery and the enteric fevers. Contact carriers are those who acquire the infecting organisms from a patient but do not become clinically ill even though the organisms may have established themselves in the tissues. Latent or subclinical infection can be identifed by raised antibody titres in the serum; in outbreaks of poliomyelitis such persons may greatly outnumber the overt clinical cases in a community. Convalescent carriers are those who shed organisms for variable periods after clinical infection. There is no defined period for convalescent carriage. Studies have shown that, after an attack of diphtheria, organisms persist in the throat of the patient for a period of several weeks. After an attack of bacillary dysentery, however, the carrier state can remain for several months. Administration of antimicrobial agents is singularly ineffective in shortening the duration of carriage and in the case of intestinal infection may actually increase the duration. Much has still to be learned about the dynamics of the carrier state. There is no clear-cut line of demarcation between the end of convalescent

TABLE 6.1   Infections that may be aquired from animals, birds and fish.

Human disease	Organism	Principal sources
Anthrax	*Bacillus anthracis*	Cattle, goats, sheep
Brucellosis	*Brucella abortus, suis, melitensis*	Cattle, goats, pigs, sheep
Bacterial food infections and intoxications	Certain clostridia, salmonellae, *Staphylococcus aureus*	Cattle, pigs, poultry
Bites	*Pasteurella multocida* and Gram-negative anaerobes	Dogs, cats
Cryptococcosis	*Cryptococcus neoformans*	Cattle
Erysipeloid	*Erysipelothrix rhusiopathiae*	Fish, poultry, rodents
Lassa fever	Arenavirus	Mammals
Leptospirosis	*Leptospira canicola* and *icterohaemorrhagiae*	Dogs, pigs, rodents
Listeriosis	*Listeria monocytogenes*	Birds, mammals
Marburg disease	Marburg virus	African green monkeys
Psittacosis	*Chlamydia psittaci*	Birds (parrots and pigeons)
Q fever	*Coxiella burneti*	Cattle, goats, sheep
Rabies	Rhabdovirus	Bats, dogs and carnivores (foxes)
Relapsing fever	*Borrelia recurrentis*	Rats
Ringworm	*Microsporum canis* and *Trichophyton verrucosum*	Cats, dogs, cattle
Schistosomiasis	*Schistosoma japonicum*	Cattle, dogs, rodents
Tapeworm infection	*Taenia* spp	Cattle, pigs
Toxocariasis	*Toxocara canis* and *catis*	Dogs and cats
Toxoplasmosis	*Toxoplasma gondii*	Birds, mammals
Tuberculosis	*Mycobacterium bovis*	Cattle
Yellow fever	Togavirus	Monkeys

and the beginning of chronic carriage.

Animals are also sources of infection that may be transmitted to man; such infections are known as zoonoses. Spread of these is uaually from animal to animal with the occurrence of an occasional human infection. In these cases the human is generally an end-host and does not further spread the infection except in rare instances such as pneumonic plague.

Examples of zoonoses are given in Table 6.1.

Soil has also a role in the production of infections. This is particularly so in infections with *Clostridium tetani* and *Clostridium perfringens* in which soil is the reservoir rather than the source of infection; the source is generally the intestine of animals. Various fungi such as *Histoplasma* and *Microsporum* are also present in soil.

Incubation period

The time between delivery of an infective challenge to the host and the occurrence of the first symptom and signs of the disease is known as the incubation period, when organisms are actively multiplying in the organs and tissues. It may last for hours, days or weeks depending on the nature of the infection. The host may feel generally unwell before the symptoms appear (the prodromal period).

THE SPREAD OF INFECTIONS

There are four main routes by which a host may become infected:

(1) the respiratory tract.
(2) the alimentary tract.
(3) the skin and mucosae.
(4) the placenta.

Within these four routes infection may be spread:

(1) by direct extension, as in cellulitis.
(2) by the lymphatics as in typhoid fever.
(3) by the blood, in the plasma or in the white blood cells, as in brucellosis and tuberculosis.
(4) by nerves, as in rabies.

Spread of infections by the respiratory tract

Organisms that produce specific respiratory tract infections such as pneumonia enter the body by this route, as well as organisms that cause generalised systemic infections such as chickenpox and measles. Three main methods are recognised in the spread of respiratory tract infections: contact; direct airborne; and indirect airborne.

Contact

This can be direct or indirect. In direct contact such as

kissing, infected droplets are passed from person to person; this is an important means of spread of respiratory pathogens that are poorly viable outside the body. For example, in whooping cough the secondary attack rate in families where contact is intimate may be as high as 90 per cent, whereas in less intimate situations such as in hospital wards the secondary attack rate is much lower. In indirect contact, organisms are transferred from inanimate objects such as cups and eating utensils. It is frequently impossible to tell whether direct or indirect contact has been the means of transfer of organisms to the susceptible host.

Direct airborne spread

Droplets are expelled from the mouth in talking and coughing and to a much greater extent in sneezing, and are conveniently classified as large and small droplets. They are derived mostly from the saliva and only a proportion will be infected. Large droplets have a diameter of over 100 μm and having been expelled from the mouth fall quickly to the ground and on to surfaces and clothing. Most fall within 2 m of the person. Small droplets, less than 100 μm in diameter, constitute the main part of the droplet mass. They evaporate rapidly and become minute solid secretions with a diameter of 5–10 μm, called droplet nuclei, that may or may not contain organisms. These particles being light can remain suspended in air currents for many hours and are probably the means of spread of many virus infections.

Although droplet nuclei are considered important in the transmission of certain virus infections the role of the larger particles in producing direct airborne infection is less clear. Their importance may lie in their ability to contaminate the environment.

Indirect airborne spread

When large respiratory droplets fall from the air they land on exposed surfaces, clothing and floors and become dried particles of secretions in the dust. Some of these will be infectious secretions and if protected from sunlight organisms will remain viable for weeks or months. *Mycobacterium tuberculosis* and *Streptococcus pyogenes* are good examples of this and these organisms can be released into the air by activities such as sweeping, dusting and bedmaking. Also, when a handkerchief is shaken dried particles of potentially infectious secretions are released into the air. Very occasionally respiratory infection, for example streptococcal sore throat, can be spread by consuming contaminated food and some cases of

diphtheria have been attributed to drinking infected milk. Certain equipment used in dental hospitals and surgeries such as air turbines, water and air syringes and ultrasonic scalers represent a major infection hazard to the staff by splatter of large and small particles.

It has been argued that because of the aerosol transmission of pathogens patients with hepatitis B or any serious infection should not be treated with ultrasonic scalers or air turbines.

Airborne spread in the dental surgery

The surgery and waiting room are areas where infections may easily be spread among patients and staff for example upper respiratory tract infection and childhood viral illnesses. Dentists should be particularly aware of the risks to female patients and staff during epidemics of rubella.

Spread of infections by the alimentary tract

The intestinal diseases, cholera, bacillary dysentery, the enteric fevers, bovine tuberculosis and rotavirus enteritis are contracted when organisms are ingested, but the alimentary tract is also the route of entry of organisms such as enteroviruses, hepatitis A virus and *Brucella* spp whose effects are produced elsewhere in the body. Spread of infection may be by food, water or by the hands.

Food contamination

Food may be contaminated at source or at any stage of its manufacture, preparation or storage. Contamination at source is exemplified by the infection of milk from a cow suffering from *Brucella* infection.

In the preparation of food, such as cream cakes, trifles and processed meat, organisms from many diverse sources can produce contamination. *Staphylococcus aureus* from nose and skin of food handlers and *Salmonella* spp from hands, rodents and flies are but two examples. The symptomless carrier of salmonellae who is also a food handler is a dangerous source of infection. Milk is another potential danger particularly if it is not pasteurised. The individual runs the risk of infection by organisms such as *Brucella abortus*, salmonellae, campylobacter, staphylococci and *Coxiella burneti*.

Water contamination

Infections may result from drinking water contaminated by urine or faeces. The nature of the drink is important; for example the ingestion of a highly alkaline drink may interfere with the protective action of the gastric juice. In most areas of Europe piped-water supplies have largely abolished water-borne infections though there is a risk in areas not yet within reach of a public supply. Classical Asiatic cholera and typhoid fever are associated with transmission by water. The Aberdeen typhoid outbreak in 1964, although disseminated by contaminated canned corned beef, was really an example of a waterborne infection because water, used in cooling the cans after their sterilisation, was polluted with sewage. Several cans were improperly sealed, resulting in the contamination of the meat.

Spread of infection by hands

This type of spread is the result of inadequate personal hygiene and the source is usually a carrier who contaminates his hands at defaecation; even a wad of several sheets of toilet paper may not be a barrier to organisms gaining access to the hands. Carriers contaminate toilet chains, wash basins, towels and door handles with their hands and infection is transmitted to another person who puts fingers to his mouth after handling contaminated articles. This is probably the means of spread of bacillary dysentery and poliomyelitis.

Spread of infections through the skin and mucosae

Simple contact

Some infections can be contracted through the skin and mucosae, for example the sexually transmitted diseases syphilis, gonorrhoea and lymphogranuloma venereum. Infection with herpes simplex is also spread by simple contact. The common wart, impetigo and ringworm can be similarly spread either by direct contact with the infected person or indirectly by contact with his clothing.

Contamination of wounds

A wound is taken as any breach of the surface of the skin and mucosae. Wounds resulting from trauma may be colonised by *Clostridium tetani* and *Clostridium perfringens* spores particularly if contaminated by earth or dust. Abrasions and pricks by rose thorns can be similarly infected. Wound infections are sometimes an occupational hazard when accidental breaches of the skin become contaminated with organisms from whatever is being handled. Thus farmers, butchers and slaughterhousemen are liable to infection with organisms of animal origin.

Implantation of oral organisms into abrasions of the skin of a dentist's hand may also lead to infection.

Sepsis of surgical wounds is one of the major infection problems of present-day hospitals and the causes of this are legion. A surgical wound is susceptible to infection from the moment of incision until it is completely healed and it is therefore exposed both in the operating theatre and in the ward. Operative and other surgical procedures, dressing techniques, environmental contamination and human factors are all implicated in hospital cross infection. Endogenous infection of wounds is also of major importance.

Injection

Injection of organisms can result from medical injections and animal or insect bites.

Medical injection procedures, including blood transfusion, immunisation, prophylactic and therapeutic procedures, are seldom involved in the production of infection, although there is a very real risk of transmitting hepatitis B by using needles contaminated with human blood. Types of injection are named according to the level of penetration, for example intradermal, subcutaneous, intramuscular and intravenous. Outwith the medical field severe septicaemia can be caused in drug addicts who make up their preparation for injection with unsterile water and often use dirty and shared needles. A wide variety of organisms, including those of faecal origin, have been isolated from drug addicts so infected. Some studies have shown that the rubber seal of local anaesthetic cartridges used in dentistry are often contaminated, and so individually-wrapped, sterile cartridges have been recommended. This is a reasonable precaution as many mandibular 'block' anaesthetics are known to penetrate blood vessels when the injection is being administered.

Animal bites. Rabies and rat-bite fever are examples of infections introduced by animal bites, but many other organisms whose sources are animals can set up infections if the bite introduces them in sufficiently high numbers and if suitable conditions for multiplication are present. *Pasteurella* spp and Gram-negative anaerobes are examples of these.

Insect bites. Arthropods are important vectors of disease such as malaria, yellow fever and plague.

Table 6.2 indicates some vectors involved in the spread of disease to man.

TABLE 6.2. Vectors of disease

Fleas	:	Bubonic plague
Lice	:	Epidemic typhus
Mites	:	Rickettsial pox; scrub typhus
Mosquitoes	:	Many infections including dengue, malaria and yellow fever
Ticks	:	African relapsing fever

Spread of infections across the placenta

An uncommon route of spread, the only bacterial infection in which this has been clearly established is syphilis in which the infected mother transmits *Treponema pallidum*. Transplacental spread is more common in certain viral diseases, notably rubella, hepatitis B and cytomegalovirus infection. Toxoplasma infection also occurs in this way.

Patterns of spread of infection

There are several basic patterns of spread of infection shown in Fig. 6.1.

INFECTION IN THE COMMUNITY

Infections in humans may be endemic, epidemic or pandemic.

Endemic infections are those occurring relatively constantly in a small proportion of the community and in the U.K. bacillary dysentery, streptococcal sore throat and measles are good examples of this. The endemic nature of infectious diseases depends on general factors such as social and economic conditions, on environmental factors such as population density and movement, standards of hygiene and sanitation, and on general herd immunity. Herd immunity can be maintained by immunisation procedures, as for example with measles, but clinical and subclinical infections are also important factors. *Exotic* infections are those that occur in endemic fashion and can be attributed

Pattern 1: No carriers
Patient→Patient→Patient
Examples: Measles
Whooping cough

Pattern 2: Carrier→Patient→Patient
↓
Carrier

Examples: Typhoid and Paratyphoid, Bacillary dysentery

Pattern 3: Endogenous infection
Healthy carrier→self infection
Examples: Skin sepsis
Urinary tract infection
Dental caries

Pattern 4: Zoonoses
Infected animal→Human patient
Examples: Anthrax, Rabies

Pattern 5: Contaminated→Human patient
soil
Examples: Tetanus
Gas gangrene

FIG. 6.1. Patterns of spread of infection.

to introduction of the disease from other countries. Cholera in the U.K. is such an example.

Epidemic infections involve large numbers of people in a community or area and result from any significant increase in the incidence of endemic infections. Many present-day epidemics particularly of virus infections such as influenza and measles are periodic. This periodicity is partly accounted for by an increase in the number of susceptible persons in the community and the contagiousness of the virus. Infection occurs when herd immunity wanes. Epidemics may also be caused by a breakdown in hygiene, a change in the virulence of existing organisms, or the introduction to the community of a new organism as in Fiji in 1875 when the island's first epidemic of measles caused 20 000 deaths.

An epidemic that has reached worldwide proportions is described as a *pandemic*, for example the Asian influenza pandemic of 1957, and becomes a national or international rather than a community problem. Such outbreaks spread quickly from country to country.

THE CONTROL OF SPREAD OF INFECTIONS

General principles involved are:

Isolation or eradication of source

Isolation measures are useful in both humans and animals with clinical or suspected infections. Eradication of many bacterial infections is possible by the use of antimicrobial drugs.

Blocking routes of spread

To control airborne infection is difficult although adequate ventilation of rooms and avoidance of overcrowding at times when respiratory diseases are prevalent may have some value. Positive pressure ventilation in operating theatres, in isolation units and treatment rooms, has proved useful.

In the control of gastrointestinal diseases many measures can be taken, including maintaining purity of water supplies; ensuring pasteurisation of milk; paying strict attention to hygiene in the preparation and handling of food, together with bacteriological monitoring of food handlers and ensuring effective disposal of excreta. Close checks until cases are free from organisms are mandatory.

Protection of susceptible individuals

Immunisation procedures have proved highly successful in the control of infections such as smallpox, poliomyelitis, diphtheria and tetanus. The administration of antimicrobial drugs may occasionally be useful in preventing certain infections in particularly susceptible individuals, for example the use of phenoxymethyl penicillin in the prevention of second attacks of rheumatic fever in children and adolescents. Antibiotics are useful in the prophylaxis of infective endocarditis in susceptible persons undergoing dental or surgical procedures. Great caution must be exercised however in administering antimicrobial drugs in the absence of firm bacteriological indications. Many surgeons now use prophylactic antibiotics before lower abdominal surgery or before major surgery in a site with substantial indigenous flora.

FURTHER READING

Burnet F.M. (1962) *Natural History of Infectious Diseases.* Cambridge: Cambridge University Press.

Duguid J.P., Marmion B.P. & Swain R.H.A. (1978) *Mackie and McCartney, Medical Microbiology,* 13th Edition. Edinburgh: Churchill Livingstone.

Dubos R.J. & Hirsch J.G. (1965) *Bacterial and Mycotic Infections of Man,* 4th Edition. London: Pitman.

CHAPTER 7

Immunity

Various mechanisms protect the individual from infection. Some are non-specific such as the secretion of mucus in the upper respiratory tract, the high acidity of the gastric juice and vagina and the peristaltic activity of the gut, whereas others such as the formation of antibodies against pathogens are specific.

The non-specific immune system

The mammalian host possesses a variety of defence mechanisms against microorganisms that do not require specific induction. Such mechanisms are collectively referred to as innate immunity.

Susceptibility to certain infections may be genetically determined. This is illustrated by the marked differences in susceptibility between species and individuals to infecting microorganisms. Man is immune to many animal infections and *vice versa*. *Salmonella typhi* produces a serious infection in man and *Salmonella typhimurium* causes a mild localised intestinal infection whereas in mice the more serious disease is caused by *Salmonella typhimurium*. Pathogenicity of certain microorganisms for a particular species has been shown in some cases to depend on the presence of receptors on host cells. Thus poliovirus can only enter and infect human cells; other determinants of species specificity remain to be investigated. Some differences exist in the susceptibility of certain ethnic groups to infection. Indians and Chinese races are more susceptible to tuberculosis than Caucasians. At the level of the individual further differences in susceptibility to infection are well known, for example to recurrences of herpes virus infection. Natural selection may play an important role in determining the differences within a species. Nutritional and hormonal factors and age also have to be considered in any analysis of innate immunity.

Non-specific defence mechanisms serve to prevent deep invasion of microorganisms and to maintain a balanced normal flora on the body surfaces. Intact skin and mucous membranes provide an effective barrier to invasion, enhanced by the constant shedding of surface cells with their attached microorganisms. Skin secretions control bacterial growth by the low pH of sweat and the antibacterial action of fatty acids. Many body fluids such as tears and nasal secretions contain the enzyme lysozyme that can lyse Gram-positive bacteria. Interferon is a substance produced by cells when infected by a virus and this acts to inhibit viral multiplication in neighbouring cells.

In the respiratory tract microorganisms become trapped in mucus and are removed by the action of cilia. The flow of body fluids such as urine and saliva has an important cleansing action as does the voiding of faeces. Gastric secretions have a low pH which kills many ingested microorganisms.

A balanced normal flora is an important aspect of immunity and this is achieved by interactions between microorganisms themselves and also with the host. This is vividly illustrated by considering dental plaque (Chap. 13). The normal flora competes with pathogens for nutrients and attachment sites on body surfaces, thus reducing the likelihood of a foreign microorganism becoming established and multiplying sufficiently to cause ill effects in the host.

When bacteria successfully penetrate these surface barriers and gain access to the tissues an inflammatory response by the host usually ensues. This involves initial vasodilatation, exudation of fluid through the now permeable capillaries and diapedesis of phagocytic blood leucocytes. The response is mediated by substances that are released in tissues following damage or contact with microorganisms. Such mediators of inflammation include histamine, kinins and prostaglandins. They are also able to stimulate pain-sensitive nerve endings, thus establishing the clinical picture of inflammation as a hot, red, painful swelling. Bacteria, their products and the mediators of inflammation, all attract phagocytes to the site; this directed movement of cells is termed chemotaxis.

Phagocytes can recognise, bind and ingest a variety of microorganisms and other foreign material in a non-specific manner but in vertebrates their activity can be rendered more specific by interaction with the specific immune system (see below). There are two main types of phagocytes in the body.

(1) polymorphonuclear leucocytes (neutrophil phagocytes or polymorphs); and

(2) macrophages.

Polymorphs comprise 40–60 per cent of white blood cells and leave the bloodstream to become the most important phagocytic cells at the site of acute inflammation. Macrophages constitute approximately 5 per cent of white blood cells and in the bloodstream they are called monocytes. These monocytes leave the blood and migrate into the tissues at a constant rate where they become tissue macrophages. Tissue macrophages are found in all connective tissues and in large numbers in lymph nodes, spleen and liver (Kupffer cells). These organs thus become important filters for foreign material carried in lymph and blood. Macrophages are the phagocytes of chronic inflammation.

Phagocytosis occurs when contact between phagocyte and particle takes place. The particle is enclosed in a vacuole or phagosome as the cell surrounds the particle; the phagosome then fuses with a lysosome in the phagocyte. Following phagocytosis a burst of respiratory activity occurs which results in the formation of toxic intermediates of oxygen metabolism. This includes hydrogen peroxide which in conjunction with halide and myeloperoxidase forms a powerful microbicidal system in polymorphs. Digestive enzymes in the lysosome then digest the microorganism. Many phagocytes may be killed by bacterial toxins during an inflammatory response. The accumulation of phagocytosing and dead leucocytes forms pus. Some microorganisms owe their pathogenic potential to their evasion of or survival of phagocytosis (Chap. 8).

An appreciation of the importance of non-specific immunity is gained when the consequences of its failure are considered. Examples include serious infections following the loss of skin in burns, chest infections following the loss of ciliated epithelium in chronic bronchitis and colitis following therapy with broad-spectrum antibiotics which kill the normal flora.

The specific immune system

A sophisticated specific immune system is found in birds and mammals in addition to non-specific immune responses. The specific immune system is characterised by a finely-tuned specificity and immunological memory. It can distinguish between self and non-self and has the built-in ability to respond in a precise manner to about 10^7 different kinds of foreign material and antigens. The cells involved in this response are the lymphocytes and each lymphocyte can respond to only one antigen. On second and subsequent encounters with an antigen the immune system responds more rapidly and with greater precision, a function of the immunological memory. The immune system deals efficiently with invading microorganisms and abnormal body cells (for example virally infected or malignant) and prevents reinfection.

Cells and tissues of the immune system

Lymphocytes are divided into B-cells and T-cells. Both are derived from stem cells in the bone marrow. T-cells mature in the thymus and B-cells mature in the foetal liver and later in the bone marrow, although their designation 'B' arises from the fact that in birds B-cells mature in the bursa of Fabricius. B-cells and T-cells carry specific receptors on their surface for foreign antigen. B-cells give rise to plasma cells that secrete antibodies in response to foreign antigens. T-cells fall into four subclasses. Two of these regulate the function of B-cells as well as other T-cells; these are T-helper cells (Th) and T-suppressor cells (Ts). The remaining subclasses have direct effector functions:

(1) cytoxic T-cells (Tc) kill foreign cells such as found in a tissue graft, virally infected cells or malignant cells; and

(2) T-cells are involved in delayed-type hypersensitivity (Td).

The latter respond to antigen by secreting lymphokines and are involved in the chronic inflammatory response and immunity to infections with intracellular pathogens such as *Mycobacterium tuberculosis*.

The specific immune response also involves macrophages which are essential to the induction of the response and are also the effector cells in the T-cell mediated response to intracellular pathogens. Macrophages and polymorphs act as phagocytes in antibody-mediated responses. Basophilic leucocytes are involved in hypersensitivity reactions and eosinophilic leucocytes are effector cells in the immunity to parasites.

The main organs of the system are the spleen and lymph nodes which essentially screen the blood for foreign antigens. In addition there are accumulations of lymphoid tissue throughout the gastro-intestinal tract, tonsils, Peyer's patches, appendix, and there are also scattered lymphocytes in the mucosae. This gut-associated lymphoid tissue (GALT) is located at the portals of entry for microorganisms. Cells of the immune system circulate in the blood; macrophages and lymphocytes also circulate in the lymph. Circulation of cells imparts a surveying function of foreign antigens, a distribution of information and a movement of active cells throughout the immune system.

Immunoglobulins and other soluble mediators

Immunoglobulins

Antibodies or immunoglobulins are secreted by plasma cells. An antibody consists of four polypeptide chains, two heavy and two light chains that are connected by disulphide bridges (Fig. 7.1). Each heavy chain and light chain is composed of a constant region and a variable region. The variable region is unique to an antibody of a particular specificity and is carried at the Fab portion of the molecule; this is the portion that binds to the antigen. Part of the constant region of the two heavy chains forms the Fc region. Differences in the Fc portion of the molecule divide immunoglobulins into 5 main classes: IgG, IgM, IgA, IgE and IgD. (Fig. 7.2). IgG is the main circulating antibody. IgM is a pentamer of the basic

immunoglobulin structure and is the antibody first found in response to a new antigen and is the only antibody that can be formed at birth. IgA is a dimer of the basic immunoglobulin structure when found in body secretions such as saliva. It forms the major antibody class in saliva, the gastrointestinal and respiratory tracts and in milk. It is often referred to as secretory antibody; in the blood IgA is usually found in its monomeric form. IgE is involved in allergic responses and IgD, produced only in very small amounts, has no direct immune function. The Fc portion of these immunoglobulin molecules can bind to specific receptors on phagocytes as well as to the first component of the complement sequence and thus can trigger various immune effector functions.

Complement

The complement system consists of nine plasma proteins that take part in a chain reaction, as well as several regulating proteins. The reaction cascade can be activated either by antibody which has bound antigen (the classical pathway) or directly by the action of some bacteria and viruses on the third component of the complement system (the alternative pathway). Activation of complement gives rise to various active substances that take part in mediating acute inflammation, attract polymorphs through chemotaxis, aid phagocytosis (opsonisation) and lyse cells and some bacteria.

Lymphokines

These mediator substances are not in themselves specific for antigens. They are secreted by Td-cells in response to antigen and thus their production is initiated by an antigen-specific step. Lymphokines are mediators of chronic inflammation and they include factors:

    (1) that attract lymphocytes and stimulate their metabolism and mitosis.

    (2) that are toxic for other cells.

    (3) that attract macrophages.

    (4) that prevent their migration from the site.

    (5) that activate their antimicrobial and cytotoxic mechanisms.

Macrophages that have been exposed to lymphokines become capable of killing intracellular pathogens such as viruses and mycobacteria, as well as malignant cells. One type of interferon also belongs to the group of lymphokines. Apart from their effect on viruses, interferons can also influence the activity of certain cells of the immune system. Transfer factor is a lymphokine that can temporarily transfer cell-mediated immunity between individuals and it has been used particularly in treating chronic candidosis.

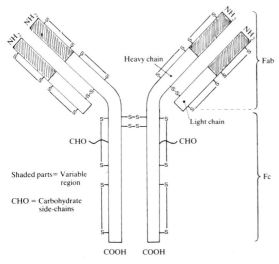

FIG. 7.1. Structure of an immunoglobulin molecule.

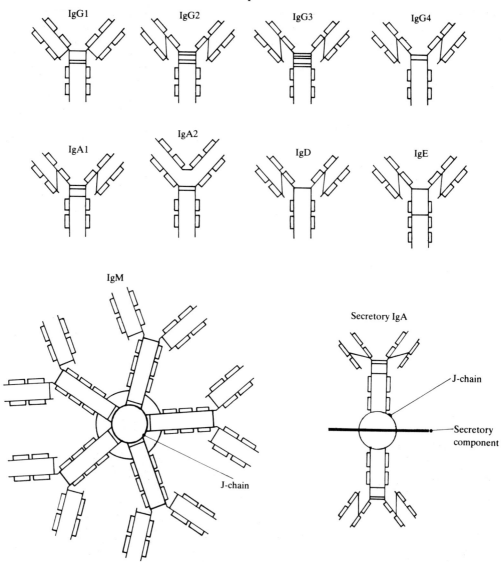

FIG. 7.2. Structure of immunoglobulin classes showing number and position of disulphide bridges.

The specific immune response

An antigen can be defined as a foreign substance that elicits a specific immune response. Substances with a molecular weight below 5000 cannot by themselves act as antigens although they may do so when bound as haptens to large carrier molecules. Most antigens are proteins or glycoproteins. Polysaccharides can also be antigenic but lipids rarely so.

Interaction of antigen with host cells

When an antigen enters the body for the first time it will encounter the very small proportion of lymphocytes (or clone) that has surface receptors specific for that antigen. Upon contact with the antigen the lymphocyte is stimulated to divide (clonal expansion) and differentiate into active cells. B-cells that carry membrane-bound immunoglobulin as receptor now start secreting IgM and mature into IgG secreting plasma cells. T-helper cells and T-suppressor cells start producing specific and non-specific helper and suppressor factors. Cytotoxic T-cells and the T-cells of delayed type hypersensitivity start secreting their various active substances. When antigen has been eliminated the effector mechanisms of the response subside but leave behind the expanded clone of differentiated cells that is ready to respond vigorously and immediately to any subsequent encounter with the same antigen. This constitutes immunological memory.

Humoral immunity

Humoral immunity is mediated by specific antibody. On initial exposure to an antigen a period of 1–2 weeks elapses before specific IgM is produced in appreciable amounts. By the third week a switch occurs to the production of IgG or, in the case of the gut-associated lympoid tissue, secretory IgA. At this time IgM disappears. Production of IgG and IgA

microorganisms to surfaces. IgA serves to reduce binding of microorganisms to mucosae. Antigen-antibody binding may also neutralise microbial toxins. The Fc portion binds to Fc receptors on phagocytes and this greatly aids phagocytosis by making it specific and more efficient (opsonisation). Contact with antigen alters the configuration of the antibody molecule in such a way that the Fc portion can react with the first component of complement, thus triggering the complement cascade which, in turn, further enhances opsonisation.

The antibody response can be illustrated by considering infection of the respiratory tract with pneumococci. This capsulate microorganism is protected from non-specific phagocytosis but it soon

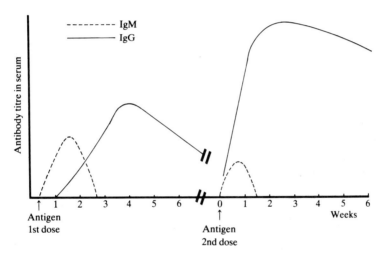

FIG. 7.3. Primary and secondary antibody response.

reaches a peak after one month and then declines over the next few weeks. Low, but still measurable levels remain for years to indicate the previous infection and the persistence of specific immunity. This pattern of response is known as the primary response.

Subsequent exposure to the same antigen triggers the specific memory cells remaining after the primary response. The rapid production of specific IgG or IgA within a few days is termed the secondary response and it persists at much higher levels and for longer than the primary response. Differences between the primary and secondary responses are shown in Fig. 7.3.

Immunoglobulins have several functions that enable them to combat infection. The Fab portion binds the antigen and can thus prevent the binding of viruses to their target cells or attachment of various

elicits an antibody response which then activates complement resulting in the attraction of polymorphs. The bacteria are opsonised by antibody and can no longer escape phagocytosis. Residual antibody offers protection against reinfection with the same type of organism.

Cell-mediated immunity

Cell-mediated immunity is mediated by specifically immune T-cells; cytotoxic T-cells (Tc); and T-cells of delayed type hypersensitivity (Td). Tc-cells recognise cells that carry viral antigen on the suface as foreign and then kill them. When Td-cells bind antigen they start secreting lymphokines that attract and activate macrophages.

T-cell-mediated mechanisms are active in immunity against intracellular pathogens. In viral infections cytotoxic T-cells kill virally infected cells; interferon and macrophages contribute to the elimination of the virus. Antibody is also found but is not of primary importance in recovery from viral infection. Specific antibody does, however, prevent re-infection with the same virus. In infection with intracellular bacteria such as *Mycobacterium tuberculosis* antibody offers no protection. These organisms are taken up by macrophages and can live and multiply inside them. A T-cell response is induced that leads to secretion of lymphokines with accumulation of lymphocytes and macrophages in a chronic inflammatory response with the formation of a granuloma. Macrophages become activated and kill the bacteria but some tissue destruction always occurs in a granuloma which is replaced by a fibrotic scar. On reinfection memory T-cells respond rapidly and the organisms are eliminated before they can multiply and spread to any extent.

Hypersensitivity

The immune system sometimes responds to antigens that may themselves be innocuous in a manner that may be harmful to the host. This is termed hypersensitivity or allergy. There are four types of hypersensitivity responses.

Type 1 is mediated by IgE. This immunoglobulin binds to Fc receptors on basophils and related tissue cells called mast cells. When cell-bound IgE binds antigen the release of active substances from the cells is triggered. Release of histamine, prostaglandins and leukotrienes causes vasodilatation and smooth muscle contraction. The response occurs within minutes of exposure to the antigen and lasts for almost an hour. Clinical examples include eczema, allergic rhinitis and asthma. The most severe form of type I hypersensitivity is anaphylactic shock. Antigens that can elicit type I hypersensitivity reactions include pollen, animal hair, foods and drugs such as antibiotics. IgE is probably beneficially active in immunity to parasites.

Type II involves IgG and complement-mediated lysis of cells carrying the antigen. This is the mechanism underlying some drug-induced haemolytic anaemias when the drug molecule binds as a hapten to the surface of a red blood cell.

Type III is mediated by immune complexes which are composed of several antigen and antibody molecules linked together to form a complex of a critical size. The immunoglobulin involved is IgG and the complexes lodge in or around small blood vessels

mainly in the kidneys, joints and skin. Complement is activated which attracts polymorphs. In an attempt to phagocytose the trapped complexes the polymorphs release lysosomal enzymes that cause tissue damage. Immune complexes of the critical size are formed in situations where there is relative excess of either antigen or antibody. The reaction develops in a few hours following exposure to the antigen and lasts for about one day.

This type of reaction is the mechanism underlying serum sickness following injection of serum from a different species as in passive immunisation. Glomerulonephritis following a streptococcal sore throat is caused by immune complexes containing streptococcal antigens. A short-lived excess of antigen will always occur at the beginning of an immune response, thus producing the complexes that result in the skin rash that occurs in many viral infections. It also accounts for the swollen joints seen in rubella.

Type IV hypersensitivity or delayed type hypersensitivity is mediated by an ordinary T-cell response involving lymphokines and macrophages. The response takes 24–48 hours to develop following exposure to antigen and lasts for several days. Contact allergies to metals, clothing, drugs and chemicals are mediated in this way.

Histocompatibility antigens and regulation of immune responses

Histocompatibility or transplantation antigens are a group of cell surface antigens coded for by the genes of the major histocompatibility complex that are placed together on one chromosome. As there are several gene loci and a large number of different alleles for each of them the number of combination possibilities is vast. Each individual thus has a unique set of histocompatibility antigens with the alleles inherited from each parent equally expressed (codominance). In man the set of major histocompatibility antigens is referred to as the HLA system (human leucocyte antigen). The complex can be divided into three classes of genes. Class I loci code for the major transplantation antigens. In man there are three class I loci coding for HLA-A, HLA-B and HLA-C antigens. These surface antigens are involved in the rejection of foreign graft tissue. Class I antigens are present on all nucleated cells and are also involved in the recognition by Tc-cells of virally infected cells.

Class II loci control the inherited ability to respond to any antigen (immune response genes). Some class II loci code for cell surface antigens that are found only on certain cells of the immune system and enable them to co-operate and interact during the immune response. In man HLA-D and HLA-Dr are coded for by class II loci. Class III genes control some components of the complement system.

Autoimmunity

The immune system does not normally act adversely to antigens of the host but sometimes this does happen and leads to autoimmune disease. Such diseases may affect one organ as in autoimmune thyroiditis or lead to systemic illness as in systemic lupus erythematosus or rheumatoid arthritis. Autoimmune diseases may be triggered off by an infection. Thus rheumatic fever follows infection with beta-haemolytic streptococci and it can be shown that antibody to streptococcal antigen cross-reacts with heart muscle. For many autoimmune diseases an association between disease presence and certain HLA types has been described. Such an association also exists for certain type I hypersensitivity reactions. The existence of HLA-linked immune disorders indicates the operation of immune response genes in man.

Immune deficiency states

Defects in both specific and non-specific immunity are known. These defects render the host less able to combat infection with microorganisms (Chapter 8).

Immunisation

Immunisation can be either passive or active.

Passive immunisation refers to the transfer of specific immunity from an immune to a non-immune individual by means of administering specific antibody. Passive immunisation occurs naturally in the transfer of immunoglobulin from mother to baby through the placenta and in the milk. Human serum or immunoglobulin from immune persons is used prophylactically following suspected exposure to tetanus and hepatitis B, as well as prior to travel to areas where hepatitis A is prevalent. Passive immunisation only gives short-lived protection until the given antibody has been metabolised.

In *active immunisation* specific immunity is induced by administration of microbial antigens in a harmless form. Toxoids are bacterial toxins that have been treated with heat or formaldehyde to render them non-toxic without affecting their antigenic properties. Examples are diphtheria and tetanus vaccines. Killed organisms are commonly used and examples include pertussis, typhoid, paratyphoid and influenza vaccines. Sometimes organisms can be modified to obtain a live attenuated vaccine that can multiply in the body without giving serious symptoms. Bacille Calmette–Guérin (BCG) is the vaccine used to protect against tuberculosis. Many viral vaccines are live-attenuated, such as measles, rubella and polio. Polio vaccine is given orally and therefore induces local immunity at the portal of entry, preventing wild virus becoming established. Live vaccines must never be given to patients with defective immune mechanisms or to pregnant women. In order to obtain a good response and long-lasting immunity killed vaccines are often given in two or three doses.

Immunological memory may then be further boosted by vaccination at intervals of 5–10 years. Live viral vaccines such as measles and rubella give full protection after one dose. Table 7.1 shows the immunisation schedule in current use in the U.K. Immunisation against dental caries is discussed in Chap. 14.

IMMUNITY IN THE ORAL CAVITY

Non-specific immunity

Several factors contribute to the non-specific defences in the oral cavity. The healthy mouth has an intact mucosal barrier with a rapid production and shedding of cells. Normal dental arches with correctly positioned teeth form a relatively self-cleansing structure that limits the build-up of dental plaque in stagnation areas. Saliva flows over the mucosae to the throat where it is swallowed together with the bacteria swept off the tissues. These anatomical and physiological factors help maintain a balanced normal flora which in itself is protective against the establishment of exogenous pathogens.

Several substances secreted in saliva may have antimicrobial activity. Lysozyme breaks the peptidoglycan molecules of bacterial walls and may help control the total number of commensal organisms. Peroxidase is an enzyme found in saliva which may inhibit bacterial metabolism, but in the concentrations found it is probably not very important. Lactoferrin is a protein that reduces the iron concentration of the surroundings and has been shown to be bacteriostatic for many microorganisms.

At least as important as the flow of saliva is the flow of gingival crevice fluid through the junctional epithelium into the crevice. This has a flushing action and also serves to transport components of the complement system, phagocytes and IgG into the

TABLE 7.1   Immunisation schedule recommended by the U.K. Department of Health 1977.

Age	Vaccine	Interval	Notes
During the 1st year of life	Diph/Tet/Pert. & Oral polio vaccine. (1st dose) Diph/Tet/Pert. & Oral polio vaccine. (2nd dose) Diph/Tet/Pert. & Oral polio vaccine. (3rd dose)	Preferably after an interval of 6–8 weeks Preferably after an interval of 4–6 months	The earliest age at which the 1st dose should be given is 3 months, but a better general immunological response can be expected if the 1st dose is delayed to 6 months of age
During the 2nd year of life	Measles vaccine	After an interval of not less than 3 weeks following any other live vaccine (Note 5)	Although measles vaccination can be given in the 2nd year of life delay until the age of 3 years or more will reduce the risk of occasional severe reactions to the vaccine which occur mainly in children under the age of 3 years (Note 7)
At 5 years of age or school entry	Diph/Tet & Oral polio vaccine or Diph/Tet/Polio vaccine		These may be given, if desired, at 3 years of age to children entering nursery schools, attending day nurseries or living in children's homes
Between 10 & 13 years of age	BCG vaccine		For tuberculin-negative children
All girls aged 11–13 years	Rubella vaccine	There should be an interval of not less than 3 weeks between BCG & rubella vaccination (Note 5)	All girls of this age should be offered rubella vaccine whether or not there is a past history of an attack of rubella (Note 6)
At 15–19 years of age or on leaving school	Polio vaccine (oral or inactivated) & tetanus toxoid		

NOTES

(1) The basic course of immunisation against diphtheria, pertussis, tetanus and poliomyelitis should be completed at as early an age as possible consistent with the likelihood of a good immunological response. Live measles vaccine should not be given to children below the age of 9 months, since it usually fails to immunise such children owing to the presence of maternally transmitted antibodies.

Reinforcement of immunisation against diphtheria, tetanus and poliomyelitis should be offered at about the age of first entry to school.

Further reinforcement of immunisation against tetanus and poliomyelitis should be offered at school-leaving age.

(2) Examples of timing doses of basic course of immunisation:

	1st dose	*2nd dose*	*3rd dose*
Age	3 months	5 months	9–12 months
	4 months	6 months	10–12 months
	5 months	7 months	about 12 months
	6 months	8 months	about 12–14 months
	Interval	*Interval*	
	6–8 weeks	4–6 months	

(3) The desirable commencing age for immunisation is 6 months of age because (1) before this age the antibody response may be reduced by the presence of maternal antibody (2) the child's antibody-forming mechanism is immature in the early months of life, and (3) severe reactions to pertussis vaccine are less common in children over 6 months old than at 3 months of age.

(4) If no immunisation has been given before school entry, the full basic course of diphtheria, tetanus and poliomyelitis immunisation but not pertussis immunisation should be given at school entry.

(5) An interval of not less than three weeks should normally be allowed to elapse between the administration of any two live vaccines whichever is given first.

TABLE 7.1 *Contd.*

(6) Although it is known from serological studies that over 60 per cent of girls aged 11–13 years have rubella antibodies, in view of diagnostic difficulties a previous history of an attack of rubella should not be accepted as a reliable indication of immunity to the disease. All girls of this age should therefore be offered rubella vaccination whether or not there is a past history of an attack of the disease.

(7) It is important to ensure that all susceptible children from the age of 3 years to puberty should be offered vaccination against measles. Particular attention should be directed to the following groups at special risk:
    (a) children from the age of 1 year upwards in residential care.
    (b) children before entry to a nursery school or other establishment accepting children for day care.
    (c) children with serious physical incapacity who are likely to develop severe illness as a result of natural measles virus infection.

---

mouth. Polymorphs and macrophages are found in the gingival crevice where they appear capable of normal function. Most phagocytes in saliva are polymorphs and although their role is not certain it appears that they have limited phagocytic function and are dying cells.

The specific immune response

Tissues. The oral lymphoid tissues are: the tonsils of the soft palate, pharynx and tongue; extra oral and salivary lymph nodes; scattered submucosal lymphoid tissue; and gingival lymphocytes which surround and protect the portals of entry into the body.

Immunoglobulins and other soluble mediators. The dominant immunoglobulin in the mouth is secretory IgA with smaller amounts of IgG. Secretory IgA is secreted mainly by the salivary lymphoid tissue. IgG is the most abundant immunoglobulin in the gingival crevice and is produced by the gingival crevice lymphoid tissue. Smaller amounts of IgA and IgM are also found.

Several components of the complement system have been detected in the gingival crevice fluid, especially the third, fourth and fifth components, but complement is almost absent from saliva.

Immune responses in the mouth. In saliva the principal component of the immune response is secretory IgA, consequently the mucosal surfaces are specifically protected by this antibody. Cell-mediated immunity and phagocytosis are not particularly important in these tissues. Viruses are neutralised by secretory IgA, which also renders harmless many food antigens. In binding to microorganisms this antibody prevents their attachment to receptors on the mucosal surface and allows them to be swallowed.

In the gingival crevice area the presence of antibody, complement, phagocytes and lymphocytes allows for many complex immunological interactions. Humoral and cell-mediated responses probably occur in relation to dental plaque antigens. Dental plaque and the host response to it are important in the understanding of periodontal disease (Chaps. 13 and 14).

Hypersensitivity reactions have been implicated in periodontal disease (Chap. 14). They also occur sometimes after administration of drugs especially antibiotics for the treatment of oral lesions.

Autoimmunity. A number of autoimmune conditions are manifest in the mouth: systemic lupus erythematosus; rheumatoid arthritis; Sjögren's syndrome; and pemphigus vulgaris. There is good evidence to suppose that some types of recurrent oral ulceration are autoimmune in aetiology. Autoimmune disease, or more frequently its treatment, may lead to oral infection, especially with *Candida albicans*. Details of these conditions can be found in texts of oral medicine and oral immunology.

Immune deficiency states. The mouth is often a site of infection in immunocompromised patients. Viruses, yeasts and fungi as well as bacteria can all be involved and infections are often caused by opportunistic pathogens (Chap. 8). Mild to quite severe infection may be present but whatever the severity treatment is usually ineffective until some correction of the underlying condition has been achieved.

FURTHER READING

Dolby A.E., Walker D.M. & Matthews N. (1981) *Introduction to Oral Immunology*, London: Edward Arnold.

Genko R.J. & Mergenhagen S.J. (1982) *Host-Parasite Interactions in Periodontal Disease*. Washington: American Society for Microbiology.

Roitt I.M. & Lehner T. (1983) *Immunology of Oral Diseases*, 2nd Edition, Oxford: Blackwell Scientific Publications.

Weir D.M. (1977) *Immunology - an Outline for Students of Medicine and Biology*, 4th Edition, Edinburgh: Churchill Livingstone.

Pathogenicity

Pathogens

A pathogen is any microorganism that can cause disease. True pathogens differ from saprophytes in that they can:

(1) survive and multiply in host tissues.

(2) produce substances that are harmful to the host (for example toxins).

(3) invade host tissues.

(4) generally survive in transit from one host to another.

This is not inevitable, however, since the host may be immune to the infecting organism; there are many other factors involved in the host–pathogen relationship. Opportunist pathogens are those which do not cause infection in the normal course of events but which may infect the compromised host - the person with impaired defence mechanisms caused for example by hormonal, metabolic, malignant disease or by cytotoxic drugs. Those undergoing immunosuppressive and steroid therapy are also very susceptible to infection with a wide variety of organisms. Children born with agamma- or hypogammaglobulinaemia are very vulnerable to infections with pyogenic bacteria because of a defective humoral defence system. Interference with local defences for example, covering the hard palate with a denture will sometimes lead to a local infection such as denture stomatitis. Table 8.1 illustrates some typical infections associated with factors that compromise the host defences.

Virulence

This is a measure of the pathogenicity of the microorganism. All pathogens are endowed with some degree of virulence which depends on many factors including structural components, such as capsules, diffusible products, or a combination of these. Virulence factors are often genetically determined and slight changes in the genome may cause considerable differences in virulence of the organism for a particular host, for example capsules of pneumococci or M protein of *Streptococcus pyogenes*. The word 'virulent' is also used in a quantitative sense. Successful attempts have been made to measure the virulence of organisms in animals and the minimum lethal dose (MLD) and median lethal dose (LD50) can be calculated. The MLD is ascertained by injecting serial dilutions of the organisms and finding the smallest dose required to kill the animal. As with humans however the resistance of animals can vary to a considerable extent and the LD50, or the dose required to kill approximately 50 per cent of the group of animals, may be a more useful measure of virulence.

Infectivity

The infectivity of an organism is its pathogenic potential. This includes successful entry to the body, establishment in the vulnerable tissues and exertion of its pathogenic effects through invasiveness, toxigenicity or a combination of both. If an organism gains entry to a susceptible site it may become pathogenic whereas in other sites it may lead a commensal existence; for example, *Clostridium perfringens* may be a pathogen in wounds causing gas gangrene but is a commensal of the gut and *Streptococcus sanguis* is a pathogen on damaged heart valves but is an oral commensal.

Transmissibility of infection

There are several factors involved in the transmission

TABLE 8.1.   Association of infection with defects in the host response.

Defect/alteration in	Causes	Effects/infections
Intact surfaces, balance of microbial environment	Local irritation or foreign body, e.g. (1) dust in lungs, (2) indwelling catheters, (3) implanted prosthetic heart valves, and damaged heart valves Lymphoproliferative disorders agammaglobulinaemia hypogammaglobulinaemia Burns Antibiotic therapy Cystic fibrosis	Bacterial infections: often low-grade pathogens, local abscesses and infective foci with bacteraemic episodes Silicosis and increased predisposition to tuberculosis Chronic urinary tract infection; mixed coliform infections often resistant to antibiotics Infective endocarditis with e.g. staphylococci, yeats and viridans streptococci Chronic *Staphylococcus albus* infection *Candida albicans* infection (denture stomatitis) *Pseudomonas aeruginosa*, pneumococci and *Staphylococcus aureus* *Candida albicans* *Pseudomonas aeruginosa*, *Staphylpcoccus aureus*, *Haemophilus influenzae*
Phagocytosis, chemotaxis and complement	Myeloproliferative disorders Granulocytopaenia Malnutrition Congenital defects Corticosteroids Splenectomy and splenic malfunction	Pyogenic infections, pneumonia and fulminating bacteraemia Meningococci and *Streptococcus pneumoniae*
Specific antibody or B cells	Lymphoproliferative disorders Agammaglobulinaemia and Hypogammaglobulinaemia (primary and secondary) Splenectomy (fall in IgM) Malnutrition Nephrotic syndrome (protein loss) Cancer Viral infections (EB, measles)	*Haemophilus influenzae*, *Streptococcus pneumoniae* and meningococcal infections. Other pyogenic bacterial infections. *Giardia lamblia* Secondary bacterial infections.
Cell-mediated immunity or T cells	Congenital defects (e.g. Di George's syndrome) Hodgkin's disease Viral infections Steroids or Cushing's syndrome Burnms and uraemia Terminal cancer Malnutrion Pregnancy Diabetes	DNA viral infections (herpes, varicella zoster, cytomegalovirus) Bacterial infections mostly intracellular e.g. *Brucella*, *Listeria*, *Salmonella* and *Mycobacterium*. Fungi, e.g. *Candida*, *Cryptococcus;* Protozoa, e.g. *Toxoplasma* and *Pneumocystis carinii* and higher bacteria, e.g. *Nocardia*. Measles *Toxoplasma*, Cytomegalovirus, herpes simplex *Candida albicans* (chronic muco-cutaneous candidosis).
Whole immune system	Congenital combined immuno-deficiency (usually rapidly fatal) Immunosuppressed patients e.g. allograft recipients	DNA viruses, *Pseudomonas aeruginosa*, *Klebsiella*, *Serratia*, *Bacteroides*, *Staphylococcus*, *Toxoplasma*. *Candida*, *Cryptococcus*, *Nocardia*, *Aspergillus* etc.

of infection from the original to the new host; for example, unless a pathogen is transmitted to a new host by a route that allows access to a vulnerable area of the host, infection will not take place. Malaria cannot be transmitted by ingestion nor cholera by inhalation. The size of the infecting dose is also important because successful transmission depends on having a sufficient number of organisms present to enter the body, overcome the host resistance and become established in the tissues. The minimum infective dose varies with different microorganisms; it is very low for *Clostridium botulinum* and *Mycobacterium tuberculosis* but high for *Vibrio cholerae*. The dose of organisms required to initiate infection can be altered by certain factors such as the presence of foreign bodies in tissues.

The degree and duration of shedding of infectious material is also important and accounts for the greater infectivity of measles than mumps and mumps than rubella.

Survival of organisms

Spore-forming pathogens such as *Bacillus anthracis*, *Clostridium tetani* and *Clostridium perfrigens* are notable for their survival outside the body, but more delicate organisms and strict parasites can survive for only limited periods under normal conditions although poliovirus can survive in fomites and hepatitis B virus can survive in dried blood.

Survival of organisms in immune individuals

This is an important factor, particularly in infections such as typhoid in which the bacilli can localise in the biliary tract; related to this is the situation where persons become carriers without ever having had the clinical illness. In rabies the virus is excreted in saliva of the normal animal hosts which become carriers. Only when man, an aberrant host, is bitten by a rabid animal does the infection manifest itself in a severe form.

Survival of organisms in vectors or intermediate hosts

Bubonic plague is spread by rat fleas and a critical factor in the chain of events leading to infection of new hosts is the ability of the plague bacilli to infect the fleas. Influenza A virus may have a reservoir in pigs.

Patterns of microbial attack

Events depend largely upon the nature of the host–parasite association but the effects are essentially localised or generalised.

Localised infection

Many infections remain localised in the 'normal' host and only become generalised if the organism becomes more virulent, if the host resistance is decreased or if the microorganisms gain access to another susceptible part of the body. The staphylococcal boil or furuncle typifies the localised infection, although many other bacteria can produce local lesions. Gonococci affect the urethra and conjunctiva and Shigella organisms the intestinal mucosa. A dental abscess is an example of an infection that is usually localised but which may spread in bone or soft tissue and may spread further usually via the blood in highly susceptible individuals.

Localised infection with diffusion of toxin producing a specific 'toxic disease'

This includes the acute toxic syndromes of tetanus and diphtheria.

Localised infection with generalised symptoms and signs of toxaemia with or without microbial spread

Streptococcal sore throat and wound infections with beta-haemolytic streptococci or *Clostridium perfringens* are examples of this and in influenza there are generalised symptoms although the virus does not spread beyond the respiratory tract.

Generalised infection

Although endogenous organisms may produce transient bacteraemia without ill effect to the host, some exogenous organisms are highly invasive when they enter the body and produce a generalised infection. These may be acute, as in the case of enteric fevers, or subacute as in brucellosis, although acute episodes of the latter can occur. Poliovirus infection may be quite undetected until the central nervous system (CNS) is involved. Spread can be direct, by the blood, by lymphatics, by the CSF, or, rarely, along nerve fibres. Certain organisms have a predilection for a particular organ or type of tissue (organotropism), for example rabies virus and the CNS. Viridans streptococci have a predilection for heart valves. Circulating microorganisms are often filtered off by liver, spleen and lymph nodes and may set up infection in these tissues. Some bacterial infections are recurrent, as in some forms of tuberculosis and undulant or Malta fever caused by *Brucella melitensis*.

Endogenous infection (Chap. 6)

Toxigenicity

Bacterial toxins can be divided broadly into those secreted by bacteria during active growth, the exotoxins, and those associated with the structure of the organism such as the cell wall which are released after death or disintegration of the cell, the endotoxins. Some fungi also produce toxins that may be ingested from food on which fungi have been growing; aflatoxin in nuts is an example of this.

TABLE 8.2.   A comparison of exotoxins and endotoxins.

Exotoxin	Endotoxin
Produced by Gram-positive and Gram-negative bacteria	Produced by Gram-negative bacteria only
Protein	Lipopolysaccharide
Heat-labile	Heat-stable
Synthesised in the cytoplasm of multiplying bacteria and released from cell	Liberated from cell wall of dead or disintegrating bacteria
Converted into toxoid	Cannot be converted into toxoid
Highly specific for certain tissues	Non-specific
High potency	Low potency
Strongly antigenic	Poorly – or non-antigenic
Effectively neutralised by antitoxin	Not effectively neutralised by antitoxin

Table 8.2 represents the classical view of differentiation of bacterial toxins but is not strictly accurate. For example, protein toxins of some bacteria may be produced intracellularly as well as extracellularly during active growth and thus a new classification has been suggested, as shown in Table 8.3.

TABLE 8.3.   Classification of bacterial toxins. From Raynaud M. & Alouf J.E. (1970) *Microbial Toxins*, 1, p.67.

Group 1:	Intracytoplasmic protein toxins of Gram-negative bacteria
Group 2:	Endotoxins of cell walls of Gram-negative bacteria
Group 3:	True protein exotoxins
Group 4:	Protein toxins with both intracellular and extracellular location during logarithmic phase

Exotoxins

These are produced during active growth by several groups of Gram-positive bacteria such as *Clostridium botulinum*, *Clostridium perfringens* and *Clostridium tetani*, *Corynebacterium diphtheriae*, *Streptococcus pyogenes*, *Staphylococcus aureus* and Gram-negative bacteria such as *Shigella dysenteriae* and *Vibrio cholerae*. Many have affinities for particular tissues; for example, tetanus toxin affects the anterior columns of the spinal cord and diphtheria toxin the heart and peripheral nerve endings. Effects of toxins are local or systemic. *Vibrio cholerae* toxin produces a local effect in that it attaches to specific receptors on the epithelial cells, causing a rise in the level of cyclic adenosine monophosphate (cyclic AMP), thereby stimulating excessive secretion of water and electrolytes from the undamaged cells of the intestinal mucosa.

Exotoxins that exert their effects at a distance are produced by *Corynebacterium diphtheriae*, *Clostridium tetani* and *Streptococcus pyogenes*.

Endotoxins

These complex polysaccharide-protein-phospholipid macromolecules are associated with the cell walls of Gram-negative bacteria including *Escherichia coli*, *Proteus* spp, salmonellae, shigellae and *Bacteroides* spp. They produce many toxic effects in the body, particularly in the vascular system, causing a drastic fall in blood pressure. Endotoxins are important determinants of the virulence of Gram-negative bacteria. They are also very powerful pyrogens, possibly mediated through prostaglandins.

Endotoxic shock

Shock is often associated with a Gram-negative septicaemia related to the release of endotoxin from the bacteria in the bloodstream. Whether Gram-negative or bacteriogenic shock is synonymous with endotoxic shock is doubtful as some patients suffer gram-negative shock with no evidence of circulating endotoxin. In addition, a syndrome similar to endotoxic shock can be caused by organisms that do not possess endotoxin. There may be some overlap in the causes of bacteriogenic and endotoxic shock although separate mechanisms may operate for each; the results are clinically similar, and many clinicians use the term 'septic shock'. Some Gram-positive bacteria and viruses may also be involved in 'septic shock'.

Patients with bacteriogenic or endotoxic shock are frequently those who have undergone diagnostic or surgical procedures on the urinary tract or bowel or have an active infection such as cholecystitis. Bacteriogenic shock can also occur as an obstetric complication. Other patients such as those who have suffered burns or trauma may be similarly affected.

Endotoxins may be detected in the blood of patients after instrumentation of the urinary tract with no subsequent deleterious effects and clinical manifestations may therefore be dose-related; the dramatic effects on the vascular system may occur only after large amounts of endotoxin enter the bloodstream. One of the disastrous effects of the shock syndrome is a condition known as disseminated intravascular coagulation (DIC) in which as a result of increased capillary permeability and loss of fluid from the vascular system, the red blood cells clump together and the blood clotting mechanism is activated. The consequence of this is that the blood supply to organs such as the liver, kidney, intestine and lungs is severely impaired causing areas of cell death.

Recently a shock-like syndrome has been associated with staphylococci (toxic shock syndrome). This was initially described as originating from infected vaginal tampons but similar cases of shock associated with Gram-positive organisms have now been reported in children.

Aggressins

Some pathogenic microorganisms possess structural components for example capsules, or diffusible enzymes which contribute to the 'aggressiveness' of an organism *in vivo*. They are not truly toxic in their own right but promote the pathogenicity of the organism. Examples of aggressins are seen in Table 8.4.

Adherence

Because there are physical and chemical forces in the body that dislodge microorganisms, such as salivary flow, mastication, and the flow of urine, blood and mucus, adherence confers on microorganisms several ecological advantages over those that have no mechanisms for retention in a site. Many have an affinity or specific adhesiveness for certain sites on surfaces, whether smooth surfaces such as teeth, or cells such as pharyngeal, buccal, bladder, urethral and vaginal mucosae. Although now thought to be an important pathogenic attribute, adherence is not essential for disease production and by no means are all adherent microorganisms pathogens. On the other hand viruses are totally dependent on adherence to host cells to gain entry. Adherence factors on the bacterial cell surface are many and

TABLE 8.4. Some bacterial extracellular products that may contribute to pathogenicity.

Description	Comment
Collagenase	Breaks down collagen and therefore has a destructive effect on various tissues (*Bacteroides melaninogenicus*)
Elastase	Acts on fibrous connective tissue (*Pseudomonas aeruginosa*)
Fibrinolysin (Staphylokinase) (Streptokinase)	Breaks down protective fibrin barriers in areas of infected tissue, e.g. *Staphylococcus aureus*, *Streptococcus pyogenes*, *Bacteroides melaninogenicus*
Hyaluronidase	'Spreading factor'; acts by breaking down the intracellular hyaluronic acid that binds together cells, e.g. *Streptococcus pyogenes*
Lecithinase	Hydrolyses lecithin with resulting lysis of red blood cells and necrosis of cells, e.g. *Clostridium perfringens*
Neuraminidase	A mucinase sialidase that catalyses the hydrolysis of mucoproteins at the cell surface, e.g. *Bacteroides fragilis*, *Clostridium perfringens*, influenza virus
Capsules	Resistance to phagocytosis especially in *Streptococcus pneumoniae* and *Klebsiella* spp

Other substances produced by bacteria that may be involved in pathogenicity include amylases, coagulase, deoxyribonucleases, esterases, lipases, mucinases and proteinases.

varied and include the M-protein antigens and lipoteichoic acid (LTA) of *Streptococcus pyogenes*, the K-88 (polysaccharide) antigen of *Escherichia coli*, and the pili of gonococci. Various surface sugar molecules, or lectins, are thought to contribute to adherence in other bacteria. Adherence is selective and many microorganisms have a predilection for certain sites (Table 8.5), although this can be prevented by antibiotics and antibodies.

When bacteria adhere to cells they may either produce a toxin, as in diphtheria, or enter the cells causing their death and producing epithelial ulceration, as in bacillary dysentery. Some may penetrate further. Viruses infect the host by entering the cells following surface attachment. Insoluble glucans (dextran and mutan) produced by some oral streptococci and other oral bacteria are important in adherence to teeth. Those that can react with the glycoprotein pellicle on the tooth surface to produce polymer bridges are thought to initiate dental plaque.

TABLE 8.5. Examples of selective adherence of microorganisms to specific sites.

Organism	Site of adherence	Possible effect
Streptococcus mutans	Enamel of teeth	Dental plaque and caries
Streptococcus sanguis	Enamel of teeth	Dental plaque
Streptococcus sanguis, mutans and *mitis*	Damaged heart valves	Infective endocarditis
Streptococcus salivarius	Oral epithelium	—
Streptococcus pyogenes	Epithelium of throat	Sore throat
Enteropathogenic strains of *Escherichia coli*	Epithelium of small intestine	Diarrhoea
Vibrio cholerae	,,	Cholera
Neisseria gonorrhoeae	Urethral epithelium	Gonorrhoea
Bordetella pertussis	Respiratory tract epithelium	Whooping cough
Chlamydia trachomatis	Urethral epithelium	Non-specific urethritis
,, ,,	Conjunctivae	Conjunctivitis
Influenza virus	Respiratory tract epithelium	Influenza
Polio virus	Human gut epithelium; anterior horn cells	Poliomyelitis

Other oral commensals incapable of producing extracellular polysaccharides may then adhere to these molecules and thus indirectly to the tooth. These forces of attachment enable many bacteria to withstand the forces of mastication and salivary flow that work to detach them.

Factors that predispose to infection

Host factors

Age. The young and old are more susceptible to infection. In the infant there is only partial specific resistance to infection, depending on placental transfer of IgG and sIgA in colostrum and in the first year of life there is lack of immunological experience of microorganisms. In the old immunological responses diminish and the functional ability of the tissues is impaired leading, in the main, to respiratory and urinary tract infection. Some 'childhood' infections are more severe if contracted by adults, for example mumps, measles and varicella infections.

Genetic factors. These are sometimes ill-defined, as in the susceptibility of certain races to tuberculosis and the occurrence of rheumatic fever in twins, but there is increasing belief that the immune response is of importance. The sex of the host may be important; the death rate from whooping cough in the first year of life is much higher in females, although exposure to the disease is equal to males.

Pre-existing disease or injury. In burns or leukaemia, for example, one of the greatest threats to survival is overwhelming infection. The 'compromised host' is very susceptible to infection (Table 8.1).

Environmental factors

Nutrition has for long been known to influence infections. Malnutrition increases the severity of respiratory tract infections such as tuberculosis, whooping cough and measles. In recent wars, infections and other diseases were rife in prisoners who were deprived of proper nutrition. Little is known about why resistance should be lowered in malnutrition although protein deficiency is known to depress the cell-mediated immune response. In addition, deficiencies of certain vitamins such as A and C have a deleterious effect on mucosal barriers. Also, chewing sucrose-rich foods leads to an increase in acid-producing streptococci in the mouth and to a consequent increase in dental caries.

Climate is important; for example, respiratory tract infections are more common in the winter months in the U.K.

Animal contact. Veterinary surgeons run a high risk of brucellosis and children playing with puppies and kittens have a greater chance of contracting campylobacter, toxocara and toxoplasma infections.

Geographical factors

Infection can be devastating in a population not

TABLE 8.6.   Infections and geographical locations.

Pathogen(s)	Geographical location	Disease	Comments
Streptococcus mutans	N. America, W. Europe	Dental caries	High intake of refined carbohydrates
	India, S.E. Asia, Africa	Low incidence dental caries	Low intake of refined carbohydrates
Fusospirochaetal or Vincent's organisms	Europe, N. America	Acute ulceromembranous gingivitis (Vincent's gingivitis)	Adequate nutrition
	Africa, S.E. Asia	Cancrum oris (noma)	Possibly concurrent infection with measles virus and malnutrition
Epstein–Barr virus	Europe	Infectious mononucleosis	—
	Africa	Burkitt's lymphoma	Possibly concurrent malarial infection
Measles virus	Europe	Measles – mild to moderate in most children	Adequate nutrition
	Third world countries	Measles – often severe with high morality in children	Poor nutrition
Polio virus	Europe, N. America, Australia	Poliomyelitis	Disease of early adulthood: rare (since vaccination) but paralysis common in cases
	Africa, Central America	Poliomyelitis	Childhood disease: infection more common than in developed countries but often asymptomatic. Paralysis rare

previously exposed to a particular pathogen. The occurrence of measles in the Faroe Islands in the nineteenth century is an example of this. Oral fusospirochaetal infection causes an ulerative gingivitis in temperate areas but may cause cancrum oris in the tropics and Epstein–Barr virus causes infectious mononucleosis in temperate zones but may cause Burkitt's lymphoma in the tropics. The reasons for this are not clear but concurrent infection, lack of hygienic measures and nutritional status may play a part in the infection (Table 8.6). The lower consumption of refined carbohydrate, however, gives third world inhabitants a low incidence of dental caries.

Local factors

Some areas of the body such as the meninges, anterior chamber of the eye and joints have very poor resistance to infection. Other factors such as surgical interference, poor blood supply and the presence of foreign bodies all predispose to infection, as does static accumulation of fluid in cysts or in blocked salivary ducts.

General host responses to infection

There are many local and general alterations in the host in response to infection. These include inflammation, malaise, fever, circulatory and haematological changes. The pathogenicity of some microorganisms depends on their ability to evade host responses, as shown in Table 8.7.

TABLE 8.7. Mechanisms of avoiding the host response.

Type of mechanism	Microorganism	Mechanism mediated by
Killing phagocyte	*Staphylococcus aureus*	Leucocidin
Resistance to phagocytosis	*Streptococcus pyogenes*	'M' protein in cell wall
	Streptococcus pneumoniae	Capsule
	Klebsiella pneumoniae	"
	Haemophilus influenzae	"
	Pseudomonas aeruginosa	Surface polysaccharide slime
	Treponema pallidum	Cell wall
	Escherichia coli	O antigen
	Salmonella typhi	Vi antigen
Resistance to digestion	*Streptococcus pneumoniae*	Capsule
	Klebsiella pneumoniae	"
	Haemophilus influenzae	"
	Staphylococcus aureus	Cell wall
	Mycobacterium tuberculosis	" "
	Brucella abortus	" "
	Escherichia coli	K antigen
Multiplication within phagocytes (macrophages)	*Mycobacterium tuberculosis* *Brucella abortus*	ability to parasitise macrophage; mechanism unclear
	Herpes simplex virus Measles virus	normal mechanism of viral replication
Induction of immune tolerance	*Treponema pallidum*	Unknown
	Some human dermatophyte fungi	Unknown
Immunosuppression	*Mycobacterium leprae*	Unknown – possibly invasion of cells of the immune system
	Many viral infections, e.g. Measles, Mumps, Cytomegalovirus, EB virus	
Inaccessibility of infected site to host response	Herpes simplex	(1) Residing in nerve ganglion (2) Shed into saliva
	Cytomegalovirus	Shed into saliva
	Rubella	Division of infected cells in congenital infection
Circumvention of immunological memory	Influenza virus	Antigenic variation: replication and shedding of slightly altered virus before any antibody response occurs. Leads to a gradual change in antigenicity of virus (antigenic drift). May be more rapid in Influenza A (antigenic shift).
	Rhinovirus	Large number of different serotypes.

FURTHER READING

Ajl S.J., Ciegler A., Kadis S., Montie T.C. & Weinbaum G. (1970–72) *Microbial Toxins*, (vols I-V). London: Academic Press.

Dubos R.J. & Hirsch J.G. (1965) *Bacterial and Mycotic Infections of Man*, 4th Edition. London: Pitman.

Mims C.A. (1976) *The Pathogenesis of Infectious Disease.* London: Academic Press.

Smith H. & Pearce J.H. (1972) *Microbial Pathogenicity in Man and Animals.* Cambridge: Cambridge University Press.

Ellwood D.C., Melling J. & Rutter P. (1979) *Adhesion of Microorganisms to Surfaces.* London: Academic Press, for The Society of General Microbiology.

CHAPTER 9

Sterilisation and Disinfection

Sterilisation is an absolute term meaning the removal of all forms of living material, including bacteria, viruses, spores and fungi. Disinfection implies that most of the pathogenic microorganisms have been removed but often non-pathogens or resistant forms of pathogens remain. There can be degrees of disinfection in contrast to sterilisation which cannot be qualified by terms such as 'partially' or 'relatively'. Antiseptics are bacteriostatic agents that can be used on skin and mucosal surfaces. Many are ineffective.

Sterilisation is usually achieved with heat or radiation whereas disinfection is generally brought about by the application of chemicals. It is important to sterilise objects such as surgical instruments and materials introduced into a patient's body. Disinfection is adequate treatment for many procedures such as the cleansing of bed pans or cutlery or the working surfaces of a dental unit because although these items must not become reservoirs of infection there is no need to achieve sterility, other than in exceptional circumstances. To obtain sterility of objects unnecessarily is expensive, time-consuming and often irritating to the staff involved. A logical approach to the need for sterilisation of certain articles but only disinfection of others will greatly reduce costs and enhance staff cooperation.

STERILISATION

Before any object can be sterilised it should be rendered as clean as possible by washing. Special precautions may be required if the object is contaminated with particularly hazardous microbes such as hepatitis B virus. Heat is the most common means of sterilising and the methods of application of

TABLE 9.1. Forms of sterilisation by heat and principal uses.

Type of heat	Use
DRY	
Red heat	Microbiological loops. Incineration of used laboratory culture plates.
Hot-air oven	Many surgical and dental instruments but not fabrics or rubber.
MOIST	
Steam at 100°C on 3 consecutive days (Tyndallisation)	Some bacteriological media.
Pressurised steam (the autoclave)	Most surgical and dental instruments, fabrics and dressings (if wrapped); most microbiological media and glassware.

heat are shown in Table 9.1. It is an efficient method providing the objects are heated to and held at the appropriate temperature for a sufficient time. Removing gross debris will reduce the time required for heat penetration. Dry heat sterilises by the denaturation of protein that occurs as it dries. Moist heat coagulates protein and operates effectively at lower temperatures than dry heat.

Red heat

Except for a few laboratory instruments such as tweezers and loops this method has no widespread application. Other forms of flaming do not sterilise and are considered under disinfection (see below).

Incineration is the widely adopted method for disposal of laboratory culture plates and other infected material.

Hot-air oven

These ovens (Fig. 9.1) are widely adopted in dental surgeries but as the time for sterilisation is long much duplication of instruments is required. Ovens must not be overloaded and must not be interrupted once the cycle has commenced otherwise sterilisation may

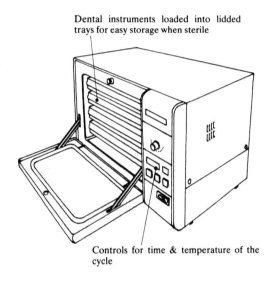

Dental instruments loaded into lidded trays for easy storage when sterile

Controls for time & temperature of the cycle

FIG. 9.1. A hot-air oven.

not be achieved. The normal operating temperature is 160°C for 1 hour or 180°C for 20 min. To this is added a heating-up time of 1–2 h and a minimum cooling period of 30 min for objects removed to a cool place. Clearly only two cycles per day are feasible in a dental surgery. Fabrics, cotton wool pledgets and paper points will all char at the temperatures in a hot-air oven. The low initial cost of this steriliser is more than outweighed by the increased cost of instruments required in the surgery but the oven adapts easily to the introduction of a 'tray system' for dental procedures.

Tyndallisation

Although vegetative organisms and most viruses are killed by boiling at 100°C for 5 min spores will survive. To sterilise some heat-sensitive bacteriological media and other objects steam above boiling water at 100°C can be used for around 30 min on three consecutive

days. This gives an opportunity for spores to germinate and then be killed on the following day's steaming.

The autoclave

Dry but saturated steam (that is, containing no water droplets) under pressure is the most efficient form of sterilisation. As the steam condenses on objects it gives up latent heat which coagulates microbial proteins very effectively. This is the principle behind

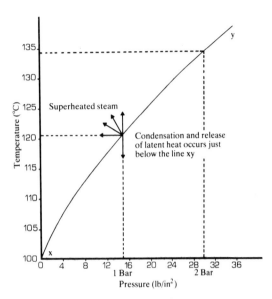

Superheated steam

Condensation and release of latent heat occurs just below the line xy

FIG. 9.2. Phase boundary of steam/water.

the development of the autoclave. The phase diagram for water and steam is shown in Fig. 9.2. Steam should be at the temperature just at the phase boundary for that pressure because above that temperature it becomes super-heated and is a poor sterilising agent, behaving more like a dry hot gas.

Water boils at 100°C at atmospheric pressure but as the pressure increases so does the temperature at which water boils. Commonly autoclaves operate at 121°C at 15lb/in^2 (1 bar) or 134 °C at 32lb/in^2 (2.2 bar). The time for sterilisation is shorter at the higher temperature; minimum accepted holding times for these examples are 15 and 3 min respectively. Taking into account the heating up, cooling and discharge times, an autoclave in a dental surgery operating at 134°C would have a cycle time of 14–15 min, whereas the cycle would be completed in 50 min at 121°C. These lower temperature autoclaves are much used in dental surgeries but models operating at 134°C and 32lb/in^2 have become available recently. The structure of a dental autoclave is shown in Fig. 9.3 and that of a hospital or laboratory autoclave in Fig. 9.4.

To be effective steam must penetrate the load to be autoclaved. All air must be removed first because mixing of air and steam produces an ineffective sterilising medium. Some autoclaves including dental ones merely displace the air by the inflow of steam. Larger autoclaves, such as found in hospital, central sterile supply departments and some microbiological laboratories, employ a pre-evacuation phase in which the air is sucked out prior to the inflow of steam thus ensuring maximum rapid penetration of the load. The inflow of dry filtered air at the end of the cycle enables dressings, drapes and other absorbent materials to be sterilised and dried for use.

Tests for autoclave function. It is important for the autoclave to function correctly with every cycle and simple indicators are available, included in the autoclave, that indicate after each cycle is completed whether the correct temperature and pressure have been obtained. A very simple check is to use autoclave tape (the Bowie–Dick autoclave tape test), which involves the penetration of steam through a wad of towels into which a card covered with diagonals of autoclave tape has been inserted. If brown lines appear on the tape this indicates adequate sterilisation. Dental trays should have a piece of tape fastened both outside and inside the lid. The tape on the outside of the lid will indicate to staff that the tray contents are sterile and the tape on the inner surface will serve as a check, when the tray is opened, that steam penetration was adequate. In an unsatisfactory run there is incomplete colour change of the tape. It is strictly only applicable to pre-vacuum autoclaves and a more accurate check on the sterilising cycle in a dental autoclave can be obtained by the use of Browne's steriliser control tubes. These small glass tubes contain an indicator that turns green when heated to the appropriate temperature for the correct time. Different grades are available for the varying sterilising cycles. They can also be obtained for hot-air oven cycles. Large hospital autoclaves are usually supplied with automatic controls or pen recorders so that the cycle can be checked in detail. Microbiological indicators of sterilisation include the use of tubes or strips containing spores of *Bacillus stearothermophilus* which are killed only at temperatures above 120°C.

Other methods of sterilisation

Radiation

Ultraviolet radiation is not an effective sterilising agent because it has poor penetration in air and, therefore, cannot be recommended. Historically it has been used to reduce the microbial counts in operating theatres and areas in laboratories where

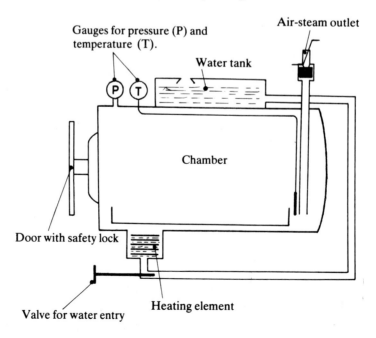

FIG. 9.3. Dental autoclave.

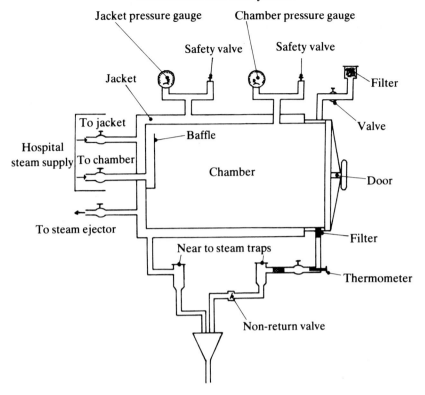

FIG. 9.4. Downward displacement hospital or laboratory autoclave.

sterile procedures such as media dispensing are carried out and it is at present commonly used in virology laboratories at the end of the day's work. Precautions have to be observed to ensure that staff are not present in rooms when ultraviolet lamps are switched on because of potential damage to skin and eye.

Gamma irradiation. This method has been adopted commercially for the large-scale sterilisation of material for clinical and laboratory use. These materials are often disposable and heat-sensitive, for example plastic Petri dishes, disposable needles and syringes. The source of irradiation, usually Cobalt 60, is lethal to all forms of microbial life.

Filtration

Many different filters of various materials and pore size exist that can be used to remove bacteria from fluids, but as they do not remove viruses they cannot be used as the sole means of sterilising a product for administration to a patient.

Air-filters usually involving electrostatic particle precipitators are sometimes used to provide clean air in areas of special risk such as some operating theatres and protective isolation suites.

Gas

Ethylene oxide gas is used for heat-sensitive products and complex equipment such as ventilators but because the gas is toxic and explodes when mixed with air it is only used in specialised hospital sterilising departments.

Formaldehyde. As a gas this is used to sterilise large spaces such as rooms or laboratory cabinets in which dangerous pathogens are present. Formaldehyde is rapidly sporicidal and virucidal but the humidity must be high for effective action and the gas is highly irritant.

Liquids

Liquid agents are best regarded as disinfectants rather than sterilising agents.

Glutaraldehyde is the only liquid agent capable of killing bacteria, spores and viruses, and it is particularly useful in killing hepatitis B virus. However, it penetrates organic matter poorly and like most liquid agents is readily denatured, deteriorating rapidly with time. It is useful for sterilising some heat-sensitive pieces of equipment and has a role in dental surgery for rendering safe such equipment especially after a patient known to have a positive test for hepatitis B surface antigen has been treated. Glutaraldehyde is used for cleansing large areas such as the floors of operating theatres if there have been patients who are high infection risks.

DISINFECTANTS AND DISINFECTION

To allow adequate disinfection an object must first be cleaned to remove organic material such as blood, pus, dentine or saliva. Occasionally organic material of high risk is treated first with strong disinfectants to render it safe before the instrument is cleaned. Usually these instruments are sterilised or disposed of safely afterwards. Methods of disinfection are given in Table 9.2.

TABLE 9.2.   Methods of disinfection.

Heat	Pasteurisation
	Boiling in water
	Flaming off alcohol
Physical	Ultrasonics
Chemical	Phenols
	Halogenic compounds
	Aldehydes
	Alcohols
	Diguanides
	Quaternary ammonium compounds
	Metallic salts
	Organic dyes

Disinfection by heat

Pasteurisation

This process is used for reducing the bacterial flora in milk and involves heating the milk to 64–66°C for 30 min or to 72°C for 15–20 sec.

Boiling water

Although boiling in water for 10 min will kill most vegetative organisms spores will survive. Boiling is adequate for disinfection of crockery and cutlery but is inadequate for dental instruments. The old-fashioned dental instrument boilers have no place in current dental or oral surgical practice.

Flaming off alcohol

Instruments can be dipped in alcohol and then passed through a flame. The alcohol ignites and burns off. Although this process is inadequate for preparing an instrument between patients it is a useful method of disinfecting root canal instruments before they are replaced in the canal.

Physical methods

Ultrasonics

Ultrasonic vibration is an efficient mechanism for disrupting microorganisms and an ultrasonic cleaning bath is an effective way of removing tooth debris from dental burs prior to autoclaving. It has been suggested that the ultrasonic scalers used in periodontal therapy have an ultrasonic disruptive effect on the subgingival microbial flora as well as an enhanced mechanical and flushing action in removing dental plaque.

Chemical disinfectants

Disinfectants usually act either by denaturing protein or lipid in the microorganism or disrupting its biosynthetic pathways. Various factors have to be considered when using any disinfectant to ensure its effective use:

(1) *Spectrum of activity*. Most bacterial spores, some viruses and mycobacteria are resistent to disinfectants. Some disinfectants are more active against Gram-positive bacteria than Gram-negative.

(2) *Rate of action*. This varies widely among disinfectants.

(3) *Microbial challenge*. Usually disinfectants are less effective against large numbers of microorganisms. Gross contamination can often safely be removed before disinfection and this helps to increase the efficiency of the disinfectant.

(4) *Moisture*. This is usually necessary for disinfection.

(5) *Presence of organic matter*. This is often deleterious to the action of disinfectants, especially hypochlorites though not to phenolic compounds. Consequently blood, serum, pus and faeces should be removed where possible. If this is hazardous initial disinfection with a phenolic disinfectant is required followed by cleaning and further sterilisation or disinfection as appropriate.

(6) *pH*. The proper function of a disinfectant is

often pH dependent, for example glutaraldehyde acts only at alkaline pH but phenols work best at acid pH.

(7) *Formulation of disinfectant.* Some agents are more effective if made up in aqueous solution; others in alcohol. A number of antiseptics are combined with cleansing agents.

(8) *Dilution.* Many agents deteriorate when diluted in water, so disinfectants should always be used in fresh dilution. Although organisms are usually killed more rapidly by higher concentrations of disinfectant it is important to use the manufacturers stated dilution. The use of a solution that is too concentrated is costly and too much dilution will reduce effectiveness.

(9) *Inactivation.* Many materials as well as organic matter inactivate disinfectants. Rubber inactivates phenols and chlorhexidine; hard water and soaps inactivate quaternary ammonium compounds. Long storage and exposure to air will also lead to deterioration of the disinfectant.

Tests of the proper functioning of liquid disinfectants

Although several tests are available to manufacturers and to specialised laboratories there is generally only a need to be concerned with 'in-use' tests. Samples should be taken from containers of used disinfectant and sent to the laboratory for determination of the viable count of bacteria, if present. Moist swabs taken from freshly disinfected surfaces may also be helpful. Sometimes bacteria such as *Pseudomonas aeruginosa* are able to multiply in diluted disinfectant and a sample from the container of 'ready-for-use' disinfectant may show up such contamination.

Examples of chemical disinfectants

Phenols

Clear phenolic solutions (Clearsol®, Hycolin® and Stericol®). These are not too irritant to skin and are suitable for gross contamination since they are not degraded by organic matter. They are poorly virucidal and are not very effectively sporicidal. Most bacteria are killed, however, and these agents are used widely in hospitals and laboratories although they are somewhat corrosive.

Black and white phenolic compounds (Jeyes' fluid® and Izal®). The black fluids are corrosive to metals and the white fluids not particularly soluble. Their smell is offensive and they are not suitable for use in dentistry.

Chloroxylenol (Dettol®). Non-irritant, this can be used as an antiseptic but its activity is poor against many bacteria and because of this it has been superseded in dental practice and in hospitals.

Hexachlorophane (Phisohex®). A useful skin antiseptic this is used as a pre-operative scrub incorporated in soap or detergents. There is some absorption through skin which has led to toxic effects in children on whom its use is now contraindicated.

Halogenic compounds

Hypochlorites (Chloros®, Domestos® and Milton®). These compounds act by releasing free chlorine. They are cheap and effective but are readily inactivated by organic matter or acid and they corrode metals. Hypochlorites are particularly effective against viruses including hepatitis B virus.

Iodine in alcohol. This is used as a preoperative skin antiseptic although skin reactions occur in some patients.

Povidone iodine (Betadine®). These agents are non-irritant, do not stain skin and are aesthetically more acceptable agents for skin antisepsis preoperatively; they are used also for surgical scrubs. Iodine kills spores as well as most bacteria and viruses. These agents have been recommended for use as anti-plaque agents but chlorhexidine is preferred for this.

Aldehydes

Formaldehyde. This is used in subatmospheric steam autoclaves which are specialised instruments developed for sterilising heat-sensitive equipment. Formaldehyde is also used for fumigation of rooms and laboratory working cabinets.

Glutaraldehyde. Less irritant than formaldehyde in solution this may still cause sensitisation in some people. It is a useful sterilising and disinfecting agent in hospitals.

Alcohols

70 per cent ethyl alcohol in water is used for preparing skin before an injection and for disinfecting clean surfaces. Isopropyl alcohol 70 per cent in water is a cheaper but equally effective alternative.

Diguanides

Chlorhexidine (Hibitane®) and picloxidine are examples of this class of disinfectant. Both are highly active against Gram-positive organisms but less so against Gram-negative organisms. Chlorhexidine is used as a skin disinfectant at a concentration of 0.5 per cent in 70 per cent alcohol and is combined with cetrimide in a commonly used antiseptic (Savlon®). A 4 per cent solution in detergent is used as a surgical scrub (Hibiscrub®) and 0.2 per cent w/w chlorhexidine gluconate in aqueous solution (Corsodyl®) is a highly effective agent for the control of dental plaque. The positively-charged molecule is attracted to the negatively-charged bacteria thus establishing a high affinity that allows the agent to be retained in the mouth long enough to be effective. Chlorhexidine also adsorbs to hydroxyapatite and to salivary mucus. Staining of the teeth and a rather unpleasant taste are significant drawbacks to the widespread acceptability of this agent but there is little doubt about its effectiveness, at least over a short period. It is therefore helpful in periodental therapy and plaque control especially in patients unable to brush their teeth effectively, for example those with orthodontic fixed appliances or interdental wiring and the mentally and physically handicapped. Chlorhexidine mouth rinses may also reduce the development of new cavities in patients with rampant caries and it is an effective addition in the treatment of oral candidosis and recurrent oral ulceration. In the latter condition it is likely that chlorhexidine controls the rapid multiplication of bacteria that occurs in the base of an ulcer where the serous exudate provides rich nutrients.

Chlorhexidine is too expensive to be used for environmental disinfection and its use should be restricted for skin and mucosae. In dentistry, however, many items requiring disinfection are made of metal which other disinfectants may corrode and chlorhexidine in alcohol is useful in these cases. Picloxidine combined with a detergent is a useful environmental disinfectant.

Quaternary ammonium compounds

These cationic detergents include cetrimide (Cetavlon®) and benzalkonium chloride (Roccal®) and are active against Gram-positive rather than Gram-negative bacteria. Their action is generally bacteriostatic rather than bactericidal, therefore they have limited use because, in addition, they are inactivated by soaps and anionic detergents.

Metallic salts

Mercury salts. These are bacteriostatic agents with poor bactericidal activity and their use in preoperative skin preparation is no longer appropriate.

Organic dyes

These include gentian violet, brilliant green, acridine and acriflavine. They have been used for disinfection of skin but their colours make them unacceptable and most have been replaced by chlorhexidine. Gentian violet is sometimes used as an astringent antiseptic for the base of oral ulcers but other treatments are almost always to be preferred.

STERILISATION AND DISINFECTION IN DENTISTRY

In dental teaching hospitals and dental or oral surgery units in general hospitals the methods of sterilisation and disinfection should be those agreed upon for the whole hospital. A disinfection policy should be established that will apply to all departments of a dental hospital. A policy is important in order to avoid unnecessary use of expensive disinfectants, the ordering of small quantities of esoteric disinfectants or use of the wrong agent. It often ensures that specialist advice has been obtained when considering the disinfection of all appropriate areas of the hospital.

Most dental hospitals and units in general hospitals will have the use of central sterile supplies in which all dirty instruments are removed from the clinic for cleaning and sterilising, packing and dispatch back to the clinic. Some additional clinic sterilisation may sometimes be required and disinfection of the fixed dental equipment will be the duty of clinic staff. In teaching hospitals it is essential to convey to the students the practical aspects of sterilisation and disinfection so that they can transfer this knowledge later to their surgeries where several surveys have shown that sterilisation and disinfection practice often falls well below an acceptable level. The realisation of the importance of blood in the spread of hepatitis B virus has at least produced a greater awareness of sterilisation and disinfection in dentistry.

In general dental practice clinic sterilisation is best achieved with an autoclave, preferably one with a rapid cycle which operates at 32 lb/in^2 (2.2 bar) and 134°C. Most dental instruments can and should be autoclaved after each patient, after having been scrubbed. Dental autoclaves are not suitable for wrapped instruments as steam penetration cannot be guaranteed. Although it is hoped that modern

TABLE 9.3. Disinfection or sterilisation of dental equipment.

Equipment	Suggested treatment	Comments
Dental handpiece	Autoclave	Use lubricant spray prior to autoclaving
Mouth mirrors, probes, tweezers, excavators, chisels, pluggers, carvers, matrix bands and holders, cartridge syringes	Autoclave	Scrub clean first
Forceps, elevators, scalpel handles, retractors and other surgical instruments	Autoclave	Scrub clean first
Endodontic files and brooches	Autoclave	May be dipped in alcohol and flamed during treatment
Periodontal scalers and surgical instruments	Autoclave	Scrub clean first
Air/water spray nozzles	Autoclave if possible or disinfect with clear phenolic or chlorhexidine in alcohol	Removable tips advised
Dental burs (steel)	Disposable	
Tungsten carbide and diamond	Treat in ultrasonic bath then autoclave	
Orthodontic bands and wires	Disposable	Use clean and discard on removal
Orthodontic pliers	Autoclave or disinfect with clear phenolic or chlorhexidine in alcohol	Autoclaving preferred; some can only be disinfected
Prosthetic trays	Autoclave	Metal trays
	Disposable	Plastic trays
Tumblers	Disposable	Plastic or paper cups
	Washing in hot water and detergent	If glass or metal
Gauzes, cotton wool and paper points	Autoclave after wrapping	Do not pack tightly and ensure autoclave has a drying phase
Linen	Autoclave surgical drapes after wrapping otherwise freshly laundered linen is satisfactory	Do not pack tightly and ensure autoclave has a drying cycle
Needles for syringe	Disposable	Never re-use
Local anaesthetic cartridge	Sterilised by manufacturer and disposable	Lightly flame disphragm before use or use individually wrapped, sterile cartridges. Never re-use
Impression compound	Disposable	Never re-use
Saliva ejectors	Disposable	Never re-use
Sutures and needles	Disposable	
Suction tips	Autoclave	
Spatulas and glass mixing slabs	Wash with hot water and detergent	If not in contact with mouth or instruments from mouth,
	OR autoclave spatula; disinfect slabs with hypochlorite	If contaminated by instruments removed from mouth
Face masks for general anaesthetic apparatus	Wipe with hypochlorite and wash in clean water before re-use	
Scrubbing brushes	Do not use routinely	Use sterile brush for surgical scrubbing
Surgery floors	Wash with detergent and dry	Daily
General working surfaces	Wash with detergent and dry	Daily
Bracket table	Wipe with chlorhexidine in alcohol or 70 per cent isopropyl alcohol in water	Between patients
Lamps	Wipe off dust	Daily. Observe manufacturer's instructions on cleaning of the reflector
Cleaning equipment (buckets, mops, cloths etc.)	Rinse and store dry	Do not store wet mops

Notes
Instruments should be scrubbed by an experienced dental nurse wearing thick rubber gloves. The instruments should be scrubbed in hot water with detergent and all traces of blood and saliva should be removed before autoclaving.

sterilisable handpieces will ensure that a sterile handpiece is used for every patient, some pieces of dental equipment pose problems; for example, the nozzles of air and water sprays often cannot be removed and are thus impossible to sterilise. In addition long lines of plastic tubing carry water to handpieces, sprays and tumblers in the modern dental unit. Such lines cannot be flushed easily with cleansing agents and consequently harbour large numbers of bacteria and doubtless some viruses for variable periods. These microorganisms are then ejected through the handpieces or water-spray nozzle when next used.

A list of items commonly found in dental surgeries with suggestions as to cleansing, disinfecting or sterilising these is given in Table 9.3.

Storage of sterile instruments

The introduction of instrument trays and lids each prepared for a particular type of treatment has greatly aided the storage of sterile instruments. The complete tray is simply transferred to a cupboard or rack from the autoclave. Instruments should never be stored in liquid disinfectants as these agents rapidly become contaminated.

Waste disposal

All sharp instruments including scalpel blades, needles and endodontic instruments should be discarded daily in thick cardboard containers specially produced for this purpose. Other waste should be placed in buckets lined with plastic bags so that they can be removed and tied up safely without the contents of the bag being handled directly.

Special problems

The patient with a transmissible infection who requires dental treatment presents the most important challenge to the protocol for sterilisation and disinfection. The protocol in Table 9.3 should be adequate for most cases and, if followed, will prevent

TABLE 9.4. Special precautions for sterilisation and disinfection after treatment of a Hepatitis B surface antigen positive (HB_sAg+) patient.

---

(1) Staff wearing thick rubber gloves should place all instruments in 2 per cent buffered glutaraldehyde for 1 h.

(2) Remove, scrub carefully and rinse, then autoclave all instruments that can be so treated.

(3) Pack all disposables and waste in stiff cardboard and incinerate directly or autoclave.

(4) Immerse all non-autoclavable instruments in 2 per cent buffered glutaraldehyde for 1 h, scub carefully and rinse.

(5) Wipe all working surfaces with 1 per cent hypochlorite solution except for metal surfaces which should be flushed with 2 per cent buffered glutaraldehyde and left for 1 h before washing off.

(6) Autoclave or incinerate gloves after the surgery has been cleaned.

---

cross-infection from an unknown carrier. Because the problem of hepatitis B virus infection has been highlighted in recent years special recommendations exist to prevent the spread of this serious disease in the dental surgery. An 'Expert Group on Hepatitis in Dentistry' was set up in the U.K. and recommended special precautions for treatment of such patients (Chap. 6) and for sterilisation and disinfection of instruments after treatment (Table 9.4).

FURTHER READING

Eccles J.D. (1980) The management of sterilisation in dental teaching hospitals. *Journal of Dentistry* **8**, 3–7.
Kellett M. & Holbrook W.P. (1980) Bacterial contamination of dental handpieces. *Journal of Dentistry* **8**, 249–53.
McEntegart M.G. & Clark A. (1973) Colonisation of dental units by water bacteria. *British Dental Journal* **134**, 140–2.
MacFarlane T.W. (1980) Sterilisation in general dental practice. *Journal of Dentistry* **8**, 13–9.
Rubbo S.D. & Gardner J.F. (1965) *A Review of Sterilisation and Disinfection*. London: Lloyd-Luke.

CHAPTER 10

Diagnosis of Infections and the Use of the Laboratory

Liaison with the Laboratory

Liaison between clinical and laboratory staff is of paramount importance in the investigation of a patient's illness and whenever there is the possibility of infection the bacteriologist, virologist or senior technician should be consulted about the laboratory investigations that should be undertaken. It is important for the clinician to give relevant information to the laboratory on the request form accompanying each specimen. Examples of information that may be important include the presentation of the patient's illness and the tentative clinical diagnosis; how long the person has been ill; whether he or she has been abroad recently; the relevant immunisation history and whether any antimicrobial therapy was given to the patient before the specimen was taken. For all specimens the date and hour of taking the specimen must be indicated.

The sooner a specimen reaches the laboratory the more reliable are the results and if specimens are important or urgent the doctor, dentist or nurse should deliver them personally. Swabs collected for virus isolation must be placed in a virological transport medium, and if a delay of more than two hours is anticipated they should be refrigerated.

Specimens

A summary of appropriate specimens for microbiological investigation is given in Table 10.1. Special precautions are required to protect some sensitive microorganisms that may die in transit. Once a specimen has been collected it is liable to desiccation, with a resulting loss of viability of organisms, particularly the more fastidious. Since anaerobic bacteria succumb to the aerobic environment of the specimen container, many anaerobic sampling and transport devices have been developed. Specimens often contain more than one organism and overgrowth of one or more may mask the presence of an important pathogen on subsequent culture. Toxic products may accumulate and nutrients may be used up in the specimen leading to death of many organisms. It is important that the proportions of different organisms in the specimen are not lost in transit and if quantitative microbiology is to be performed, as in the examination of specimens of urine, there must be no change in numbers of microorganisms before culture.

Transport media have been developed to overcome many of these hazards. They are usually liquid or semi-solid but one drawback to their use is that of dilution of the specimen; another danger is the possible feeling that a specimen in transport medium is less urgent because it is protected. Transport media often contain inhibitory substances to prevent bacterial multiplication in transit. Viral transport media and chlamydia transport media contain antibiotics which kill off most bacteria and prevent the accumulation of toxic products which may affect the virus or chlamydia. Some transport media contain charcoal powder which adsorbs toxic products. Reduced transport media such as 'Reduced Transport Fluid' protect anaerobes much more than non-reduced media. It is important to use the correct transport medium and if investigation for more than one type of microorganism is required several specimens should be taken and placed in the appropriate medium. Any collection of pus should be sent in a plain sterile container as pus is itself a most effective transport medium. Chilling is often useful in reducing the loss of microorganisms in a specimen but it should not be used for neisseriae which are sensitive to cold. Viruses will readily withstand freezing.

TABLE 10.1. Suitable specimens for microbiological investigations.

Tissue or System involved	Specimen	Comments
Skin	Swab (moisten in sterile saline if lesion is dry)	Examine for bacteria and yeasts
	Scrapings	Examine for fungi
	Vesicle fluid	Examine for viruses (electronmicroscopy and culture)
	Serum	Tests for viral infection
Hair and Nails	Clippings	Examine for fungi
Blood (bacteraemia and septicaemia)	Blood culture	Sterile precautions necessary. Multiple specimens required after consulting laboratory
	Clotted blood	Culture for *Salmonella typhi*
Urinary Tract	Mid-stream specimen of urine/supra-pubic aspirate/catheter specimen of urine (not from a collecting bag)	For quantitative and qualitative bacteriology
Gastrointestinal tract	Faeces	Culture for bacteria and viruses; toxin detection for *Clostridium difficile;* light microscopy for parasites and protozoa; electron-microscopy for viruses
	Jejunal aspirates	Culture and microscopy for bacteria and protozoa
	Serum	Serological tests for enteric fevers
Upper Respiratory Tract	Pernasal, throat and nose swabs; saliva	Culture for *Bordetella pertussis.* Culture for beta-haemolytic streptococci other bacteria and viruses
	Throat washings or nose and throat aspirates	Culture and immunofluorescence for viruses
Lower Respiratory Tract	Sputum	Culture for bacteria, viruses and fungi; fluorescent microscopy for many viruses, *Mycobacterium tuberculosis* and *Legionella*
	Serum	Serological tests for viral and fungal diseases
Meninges	Cerebrospinal fluid	Sterile precautions essential: for cell count, microscopy and culture. Analysis of lactate will help differentiate viral from bacterial meningitis. CIE may speed diagnosis (see text)
	Serum	Serological tests for viruses
	Faeces (viral meningitis)	For virus detection
Eyes	Swab	Plate directly at bedside to overcome bactericidal activity of lysozyme. For chlamydiae use chlamydia transport medium
	Smear of secretions	Heat-fix on microscope slide at bedside
Ears	Swab	Culture for bacteria and fungi
Genital Tract	Swab in Amies' or Stuart's Transport Medium	For bacterial and yeast culture and microscopy for gonococci and *Trichomonas* (wet film)
	Swabs in chlamydia and viral transport medium	Culture of chlamydia and viruses
	Smear of discharge: (1) heat fixed, (2) wet film	For detection of gonococci, for *Trichomonas*
	Serum	Serological tests for syphilis
Abscess	Pus	Aspirates preferred to swab; enables gas-liquid chromatographic analysis and culture
Wounds	Pus or swab	Avoid contamination from skin; pus preferred
	Tissue	Send small samples in dry sterile containers for homogenisation, culture and microscopy
Joints	Joint fluid	Sterile precautions essential for microscopy and culture
	Serum	Serological tests for staphylococcal and streptococcal infection and viruses
Mucosal lesions	Swab	Avoid contamination with normal flora. Use transport medium if necessary; culture for bacteria, fungi and viruses
	Smears from scraping of lesion	Prepare in clinic, heat-fix for light fluorescent microscopy; useful for gonococci and yeasts
	Serum	Serological tests for staphylococcal and streptococcal infection and viruses

Sites from which swabs or aspirates are taken should not be wiped with alcohol or disinfectant before sampling because this may kill organisms in the sample during transit. If a patient is to have antibiotics specimens should be collected first because recovery of microorganisms from specimens loaded with antibiotic is poor, even though the organism may be able to overcome the antibiotic *in vivo*. If a specimen is taken from a patient on antibiotics the laboratory should be informed in order to help in the planning of appropriate laboratory procedures or in the interpretation of results.

Specimen containers should always be sterile before use and those with broken seals should be discarded.

Specimens from the mouth

A summary of the type of specimens taken from the mouth is given in Table 10.2. Swabs are commonly taken but pus, where present, should be aspirated and sent in the syringe or a specimen bottle to the laboratory. Dry lesions, such as on perioral skin, should be sampled with a swab moistened in sterile saline. Swabs should be applied carefully to the lesion and rolled over to gather any infecting organisms on to the whole swab. Care should be taken to avoid contaminating the swab with microorganisms from other sites; this is especially difficult with swabs taken from the mouth. Samples obtained on a sharpened wooden stick or a sterile scaler can be used to produce a smear on a microscope slide, which should be heat-fixed in the clinic before being sent to the laboratory. Tongue depressors are convenient tools for scraping white lesions in the mouth without causing too much trauma. The scraping can be applied to a microscope slide and heat-fixed.

Special sampling tools are needed to collect dental

TABLE 10.2. Suitable specimens from the mouth for microbiological examination.

Lesion or site of lesion	Specimen	Comments
Facial and perioral skin	Moistened or dry swab	Culture for yeasts and bacteria
	Smear of scraping (heat-fixed)	Prepare in clinic; microscopy for yeasts
	Vesicle fluid	Culture for viruses and electronmicroscopy
	Aspiate of abscess	Gross examination (for sulphur granules); microscopy and culture
	Serum	Serological tests for viruses
Lips	Vesicle fluid	Culture for viruses and electronmicroscopy
	Serum	Serological tests for viruses and syphilis
Dorsum of tongue	Swab	Culture for yeasts and bacteria
	Smear of scraping (heat-fixed)	Prepare in clinic; microscopy for yeasts and bacteria
Other mucosal surfaces	Swab	Culture for bacteria, yeasts and viruses
	Smear of scraping (heat-fixed)	Microscopy for yeasts and bacteria
	Vesicle fluid	Culture for viruses and electronmicroscopy
	Biopsy tissue	Culture for bacteria and viruses; microscopy for yeasts and suspected tuberculosis
	Serum	Serological tests for viruses
Dental abscess or suspected infected cyst	Aspirate	Culture for bacteria
Infected root canal	Paper point or barbed brooch	Avoid contamination; use semi-solid transport medium. For semi-quantitative culture
Carious tooth	Tooth	As yet of no diagnostic or prognostic value but research into carious lesions involves a variety of sampling procedures
Dental plaque	Scraping	As yet of no diagnostic or prognostic value but research into dental plaque involves a variety of sampling tools and procedures
Gingivae and gingival crevice	Scraping on a sharpened woodstick or sterile scaler	Culture not likely to yield much of value in diagnosis. Smear can be diagnostic for infection with Vincent's organisms (fusospirochaetal infection) and viral culture is possible.
	Serum	Serological tests for viruses

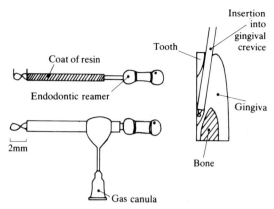

FIG. 10.1. Device for sampling from the gingival crevice. To avoid contamination from the more superficial areas of the crevice the reamer is retracted into the resin coat prior to removal. Oxygen-free gas passes through the canula to keep the sample reduced prior to inoculation of media. (Courtesy of Dr J. M. Hardie).

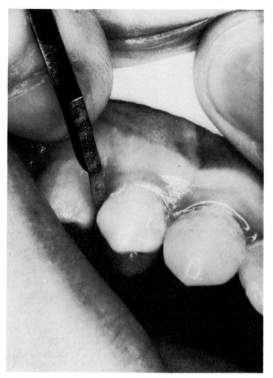

FIG. 10.3. The device shown in Fig. 10.2. in use (Courtesy of Dr J. M. Hardie).

plaque from approximal regions and from the gingival crevice. These tools usually involve a hollow needle into which is inserted a thin abraded wire or endodontic brooch. The needle is placed in the site and the wire pushed through to collect an uncontaminated sample. The wire is then retracted into the needle prior to removal from the mouth. Some variations include a supply of oxygen free gas to protect the anaerobic bacteria in the sample (Figs. 10.1, 10.2 and 10.3).

Endodontic specimens are usually collected on a paper point or barbed brooch. This may be protected by a surrounding sleeve that engages the opening of the root canal.

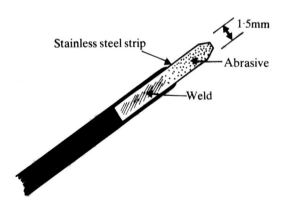

FIG. 10.2. Device for sampling approximal dental plaque (Courtesy of Dr J. M. Hardie).

Diagnostic approaches in microbiology

The objects of diagnostic microbiology are two-fold; firstly, to identify the causative organisms of infection in the patient and, secondly, to establish whether the results of infection, namely antibodies, are present in the patient's serum. Before an organism can be accepted as the cause of an infection certain criteria, known as the Koch-Henle postulates, must be satisfied. These state that the organism must be present in the host and be able to be isolated in pure culture from the infected lesions; that the infection can be reproduced when the organism from the pure culture is inoculated into a susceptible species; and that the organism can be re-isolated during the course of the experimental disease. These postulates are now supplemented by demonstration of an increase in the antibody titre to the infecting organism during the course of the disease. The Koch-Henle postulates cannot be fulfilled for some diseases including leprosy because the organisms that are considered to be the cause of the disease cannot be cultured. Also, the same organism can cause several different syndromes and several organisms can produce similar syndromes.

The commensal flora of the various areas of the body introduces practical problems in attempts to identify the causes of endogenous infection and this has considerable relevance to investigations of the microbial causes of dental caries and periodontal disease. Their antibody responses are complex and although there is little doubt about the close relationship with microorganisms the Koch-Henle postulates have not yet been' satisfied for these diseases.

faeces for cysts and parasites and vaginal exudates for trichomonads. Fixed films are routinely made in the examination of sputum, urine and wound swabs and are commonly stained by Gram's method; they reveal the presence of pus cells, red blood cells and organisms. Other stains can be used such as the Ziehl-Neelsen for tubercle bacilli, Albert's for corynebacteria and methyl violet for Vincent's organisms. In the examination of skin lesions, faeces and throat swabs the Gram film may not be helpful

TABLE 10.3. Serological tests used in microbiology.

Test	Use in microbiology
Precipitation	Grouping of beta-haemolytic streptococci, toxin detection in *Corynebacterium diphtheriae,* typing pneumococci and detecting antibody to some fungi.
Counterimmunoelectrophoresis	Detection of antigens to meningococci, pneumococci and *Haemophilus.*
Agglutination	Streptococcal grouping, *Salmonella* identification.
Haemagglutination	Hepatitis B surface antigen (HB_sAg) detection.
Haemagglutination inhibition	Ortho-and para-myxovirus infections, EB virus infection (Paul Bunnell Test).
Haemagglutination in cold	*Mycoplasma pneumoniae* infection.
Complement fixation test (CFT)	For viruses such as herpes and adenovirus.
Direct Fluorescent labelling	For respiratory tract viruses and gonococci.
Indirect Fluorescent labelling	*Legionella* antibodies and antibodies to many viruses.
Radioimmunoassay (RIA)	Assay of aminoglycoside antibiotics in serum, detection of HB_sAg and antibodies to HB_sAg.
Enzyme linked immunosorbent assay (ELISA)	Detection of antibody against beta-haemolytic streptococci, salmonellae and *Treponema pallidum* detection of HB_sAb. Increasingly used to detect antibody to viruses and viral antigens.

Table 10.3 contains a list of common serological tests in microbiology with examples of their uses. Textbooks of laboratory method will give details of these tests. Clinicians wishing to investigate a particular disorder should be advised by the laboratory of the types of tests available, the possible value of these tests and the specimens required.

Laboratory investigation of bacterial and fungal infection

Inspection

This includes checking that the specimen and the request form match and looking for any gross features in the specimen that may aid diagnosis, such as the presence of sulphur granules in the pus of a case of actinomycosis.

Microscopy

Direct wet films are important in the examination of

although it can indicate the appropriate method of culture. Only very occasionally can it be reasonably diagnostic, as in the demonstration of Vincent's organisms from gingival scrapings and Gram-negative intracellular diplococci from the cerebrospinal fluid of a case of meningitis.

Phase contrast microscopy is useful in the investigation of spirochaetal infections and for detecting fungal hyphae in specimens of skin or nails. Fluorescent antibody techniques are of value in the direct demonstration of organisms in clinical material, namely *Bordetella pertussis* in naso-pharyngeal swabs, *Treponema pallidum* in exudates and *Neisseria gonorrhoeae* in urethral discharge.

Culture

Growth requirements of bacteria and fungi are described in Chap. 3.

In some cases the specimen may have to be processed before culture; for example, sputum is homogenised and many fluids are centrifuged. Blood agar is a commonly used medium in medical bacteriology, but many others are available, including selective media. For example, the addition of potassium tellurite to blood agar makes the isolation of corynebacteria from a throat swab more possible by inhibiting growth of many of the throat commensals and vancomycin inhibits many Gram-positive bacteria, thus favouring the growth of *Bacteroides*. Yeasts grow at low pH and this is used in malt or Sabouraud's medium to inhibit bacteria and allow the yeasts to be isolated.

Blood agar plates may be incubated aerobically or anaerobically but frequently both methods are used. Culture plates can be incubated anaerobically in an anaerobic cabinet or in an anaerobic jar from which oxygen has been removed and replaced by a hydrogen-carbon dioxide mixture, either from a gas cylinder or by including in the jar one of the commercially-produced envelopes which produce these gases when water is added. Liquid media such as Robertson's meat broth also produce anaerobic conditions in the meat particles at the bottom of the tubes. Finally, many cultures grow better in an atmosphere of 5–10 per cent carbon dioxide, for example gonococci, oral streptococci and *Bacteroides* spp and this should be used for routine specimens. Most cultures are incubated at 37°C but yeasts are often incubated at 22–28°C.

Biochemical tests

Many bacteria produce enzymes and other substances that are characteristic of the particular organisms. These are frequently of value in the diagnostic process, for example the production of coagulase by *Staphylococcus aureus* and oxidase by *Neisseria gonorrhoeae*. The analysis by gas-liquid chromatography of the free fatty acids produced in culture is useful for the identification of some anaerobic bacteria and more particularly for the detection of anaerobes in a specimen of pus or other fluid.

Special tests applied to isolates

These include epidemiological markers such as bacteriophage typing for staphylococci, colicine production by *Shigella sonnei* and pyocine production by *Pseudomonas aeruginosa*.

Antibiotic sensitivity testing

As well as isolating and identifying microorganisms in specimens the laboratory should determine their sensitivity to appropriate antimicrobial drugs. If blind therapy is required in advance of the results of sensitivity tests the microbiologist with his knowledge of current sensitivity patterns is best equipped to advise on this.

It is sometimes important to determine the bacteriostatic and bactericidal concentrations of an antibiotic for a bacterium. This helps the clinician assess the dosage of the antibiotic and is for example, an essential part of the treatment of endocarditis caused by members of the viridans streptococci.

In such serious infections it is necessary to monitor the concentration of antibiotic in the patient's blood. Two samples are taken daily, one just before the dose of antibiotic, the 'trough' level and one 30 min to 1 h after the parenteral dose, the 'peak' level. If the antibiotic concentration falls to less than the minimum concentration of antibiotic that inhibits the organism (minimum inhibitory concentration or MIC) then treatment is ineffective. In practice it is usually necessary for trough levels of antibiotic to be two or four times greater than the MIC for the infecting organism. Peak levels should be below the threshold for toxicity to the host.

Toxic antibiotics such as the aminoglycosides are monitored daily in the same way. Peak and trough blood levels are taken and the serum is analysed by one of a variety of techniques to give a rapid evaluation of the amount of antibiotic present.

The laboratory is also well placed to keep track of the antibiotic susceptibility patterns of bacteria isolated within its catchment area. A close check should be kept on the emergence of resistance to commonly used antibiotics. This will include detecting resistance to penicillin among gonococci and the more common development of multiple drug resistance in hospital isolates of staphylococci and coliform organisms. The laboratory should advise on an appropriate policy to reduce the development or spread of antibiotic resistance.

Laboratory investigation of viral infection

Microscopy

By the use of the electron microscope a presumptive diagnosis may be made of certain virus infections. Historically the typical virons of smallpox from skin vesicles were quickly differentiated from chickenpox but electron microscopy is now used to detect rotaviruses in faeces and for examining vesicle fluid and biopsy material. The light microscope may also be useful, as in the diagnosis of rabies. In this disease inclusion bodies (Negri bodies) can be demonstrated in the cytoplasm of brain cells. Immunofluorescence is now commonly used for rapid identification of viruses in specimens and tissue culture.

Culture

Methods of culture of viruses are described in Chap. 4. Growth of viruses in tissue culture produces a cytopathic effect (CPE) which may be diagnostic. Further tests such as haemadsorption and inhibition of haemadsorption assist in the identification of the virus.

Serological tests

These are widely used to detect infection with microorganisms. They are of two types, direct for detection of antigen and indirect for detection of antibody. They are used in the diagnosis of infections caused by a wide range of bacteria, viruses and fungi (see Table 10.3).

Detection of antigen. In agglutination and precipitation tests suspensions of the organisms are tested against a range of antisera of known identity; this technique can be used to group isolates of beta-haemolytic streptococci. Hepatitis B surface antigen (HB$_s$Ag) can be detected in a specimen by a haemagglutination test. Fluorescent antibody tests can be used for the rapid detection of gonococcal antigen.

In recent years counterimmunoelectrophoresis (CIE) has been used in the detection of many antigens such as those present in meningococci, pneumococci, streptococci, salmonellae, *Haemophilus influenzae* and *Proteus* spp. This technique can provide a prompt identification of the causative organism in bacterial meningitis. Enzyme-linked immunosorbent assay (ELISA) can be used for the detection of viral antigens, e.g. rotavirus in faeces.

Detection of antibody By demonstrating serum antibodies to a suspected organism it is inferred that the patient is infected with the organism. A single test is totally inadequate because if the antibody titre is raised it is impossible to say whether this is due to past or present infection. Two tests must be performed, one at the beginning of the illness and the other 10–14 days later, and if a rising titre or level of antibodies is demonstrated between the two specimens (ideally a four-fold difference) it can be said that the patient's infection is current. It is usual to test for agglutinating antibodies, for example in the diagnosis of brucellosis, and complement-fixing antibodies as in the serological diagnosis of syphilis and many viral diseases. Other tests which have proved valuable in the detection of antibody in more recent times are radioimmunoassay (RIA) which is specific, sensitive and requires only small quantities of antigen, and enzyme-linked immunosorbent-assay (ELISA) which has been successfully used to detect antibodies against streptococci, other bacteria and many viruses. Non-specific tests are also available, including the Paul-Bunnell test for infectious mononucleosis and the Wassermann Reaction for syphilis. Indirect immunofluorescence is used to detect antibodies to EB virus.

Animal tests

In bacteriology these are used to test whether organisms such as clostridia and corynebacteria are toxigenic; they are helpful also in establishing the diagnosis of tuberculosis. They may be useful in virology, for example in the isolation of coxsackie group A viruses by intraperitoneal inoculation of suckling mice.

FURTHER READING

Cruickshank R., Duguid J.P., Marmion B.P. & Swain R.H.A. (1975) *Medical Microbiology*, Vol. II, 12th Edition. Edinburgh: Churchill Livingstone.

Duguid J.P., Marmion B.P. & Swain R.H.A. (1978) *Mackie and McCartney Medical Microbiology*, Vol. I, 13th Edition. Edinburgh: Churchill Livingstone.

Stokes E.J. & Ridgway G.L. (1980) *Clinical Bacteriology*, 5th Edition. London: Edward Arnold.

Timbury M.S. (1978) *Notes on Medical Virology*, 6th Edition. Edinburgh: Churchill Livingstone.

Tyrrell D.A.J., Phillips I., Goodwin C.S. & Blowers R. (1979) *Microbial Disease: The use of the laboratory in diagnosis, therapy and control.* London: Edward Arnold.

CHAPTER 11

Treatment of Infections:

Antibiotics and Chemotherapy

Principles of use

The choice of drug

This depends primarily on the nature of the infecting organism and its antibiotic sensitivity pattern. Antibiotics should be used on a rational bacteriological basis although there is a place for an educated guess in a clinical emergency such as septicaemia or osteomyelitis in a child. Pyrexial patients with a dental abscess may be given an antibiotic as an adjunct to drainage. The local laboratory should be able to provide information on the likely sensitivity patterns of the probable infecting organisms based on recent experience. Occasionally, as in Vincent's gingivitis, a Gram-stained smear from the lesion is diagnostic and is sufficient to indicate the appropriate antibiotic.

Specimens must be taken prior to starting treatment which should be reviewed after the pathogen has been identified and antibiotic sensitivity patterns established. Consideration must be given as to whether a bactericidal or bacteriostatic drug of broad or narrow spectrum should be used.

Bactericidal and bacteriostatic action

Antimicrobial drugs may be bactericidal and rapidly kill bacteria, or bacteriostatic and inhibit multiplication without actually killing the organisms. The line of demarcation between the two actions is not clear-cut and is dependent on factors such as the extent of the bacterial challenge, the concentration of the drug and the organism concerned; some drugs such as erythromycin are bacteriostatic at normal dosage but are bactericidal in higher concentrations. Bactericidal drugs are to be preferred to bacterio-

static drugs but a critical factor in the cure of infection is the patient's own defence system and bacteriostatic drugs may be able to inhibit multiplication of the bacteria sufficiently to allow their elimination by phagocytes.

Broad-spectrum and narrow-spectrum drugs

Broad-spectrum drugs such as the tetracyclines and ampicillin have a wide range of activity against both Gram-positive and Gram-negative bacteria, whereas flucloxacillin has a narrow spectrum. Narrow-spectrum drugs are to be preferred because of their greater specificity and unlike broad-spectrum drugs they do not have the same adverse effects on the normal flora of the body. Broad-spectrum drugs can so alter the composition of the flora at various sites that its normal protective effect is ruined, and it is well recognised that certain pathogenic organisms can colonise such areas and produce superinfection, as in infection of the mouth by *Candida* spp.

Combinations of drugs

In general a single antimicrobial drug should be used for the treatment of a particular infection but there are indications for the use of a combination of drugs. These are:

(1) to achieve a synergistic effect, the combination of drugs producing a much greater effect than either drug alone,

(2) to prevent the development of bacterial resistance,

(3) to deal with mixed infections.

Synergism is well demonstrated in the treatment of infective endocarditis caused by *Streptococcus faecalis*. It has been shown that a combination of penicillin and an aminoglycoside is often therapeutic whereas this would not be so with full doses of either drug alone. Synergism is also well demonstrated in the laboratory in the combination of sulphonamide and trimethoprim in the drug cotrimoxazole. The use of combinations of drugs to prevent the emergence of drug-resistant strains is illustrated in the treatment of tuberculosis. In this disease treatment is prolonged and resistance to single drugs occurs quickly. The incidence of mutants resistant to a single drug may be in the order of one per 10^7 cell divisions so that if two drugs are given the chances are then only one per 10^{14}.

Antibiotic prophylaxis

This area is highly controversial. There is no doubt that antibiotics are administered without proper reason in the hope that any pathogen present might be eliminated. Even if pathogenic organisms are present in a particular area of the body frequently the antibiotics given prophylactically are ineffective against these, resulting in the selection of resistant organisms.

There are however some clear and justifiable indications for long-term or short-term prophylaxis.

Short-term prophylaxis

In trauma, when there are the possibilities of tetanus or gas gangrene if the wound becomes contaminated by *Clostridium tetani* or *Clostridium perfringens*, benzyl or phenoxymethyl penicillin should be given. Following thigh amputation in the elderly there is a risk of endogenous infection from *Clostridium perfringens* and a similar policy should be followed. In certain abdominal operations where the risk of endogenous infection is high antibiotics can be given for the immediate preoperative and peroperative period. An example of this is the use of metronidazole to eliminate the anaerobic organisms that are often associated with abdominal sepsis. A striking example of short-term prophylaxis in dentistry is the administration of a penicillin prior to some dental procedures, particularly extractions, to patients at risk of developing infective endocarditis.

Long-term prophylaxis

Children who have had a primary attack of rheumatic fever run a high risk of a subsequent attack and phenoxymethyl penicillin should be given to them to prevent reinfection with *Streptococcus pyogenes*. Urinary tract infection in children, particularly girls, and in some adult women who suffer repeated attacks can be avoided by the administration of antibiotics,

such as nitrofurantoin and cotrimoxazole. In long-term prophylaxis, however, it is mandatory to check the antibiotic sensitivities of the infecting organism because of the very real risks of production of resistance.

Within these widely differing sets of circumstances there are grey areas where there can be arguments for or against prophylaxis, as in open heart surgery, before anaesthesia in patients with chronic respiratory disease and in biliary tract surgery.

General considerations in antibiotic therapy

Dosage. Antibiotics should be given in therapeutic doses. Doses should be sufficient to produce a concentration of antibiotic greater than that required to kill the organism or inhibit its growth.

Duration of treatment. This should be long enough to allow for all or nearly all the organisms to be eliminated. In most cases any organisms remaining will be dealt with by the host defence mechanisms.

Route of administration. Antibiotics must be given parenterally to seriously ill patients to overcome any problems of absorption from the intestinal tract. Oral antibiotics must be acid stable.

Distribution. The antibiotic must penetrate to the site of infection. To allow this it is often necessary to have surgical intervention, for example draining pus from 'walled-off' abscesses and removing renal stones causing obstruction with supervening sepsis in the urinary tract.

Excretion. Knowledge of the pathway of excretion of a drug can be of assistance in the treatment of certain infections. For example, nitrofurantoin and nalidixic acid are excreted in the urine and this makes them suitable for use in urinary tract infections.

Toxicity. Many drugs have side effects, the more serious being ototoxicity, nephrotoxicity and bone marrow aplasia. Hypersensitivity may also occur.

Drug incompatibility. Nalidixic acid, for example, potentiates the action of warfarin. Metronidazole taken with alcohol produces an effect similar to that of antabuse.

Local treatment. This should be carried out with antibiotics such as neomycin that are not used systemically, because if drug resistance occurs a valuable systemic drug becomes useless for treatment

TABLE 11.1.   The properties of a hypothetical wonder drug Miraclemycin (courtesy of Professor J. G. Collee).

Potently bactericidal

Cheap

Non-toxic, non-irritant, non-staining (for example, to developing tooth enamel)

Specific (narrow-spectrum)

High concentrations of active form obtainable in body fluids or tissues — especially in blood, urine, CSF, bile, bone, brain and eye

No resistance or cross-resistance

No sensitisation

No significant protein-binding

Effective orally, but absorbed proximally

Stable, but metabolised by man

---

of serious infection in that patient. No antibiotic is perfect; each has some drawback. (Properties of a hypothetical wonder drug (Miraclemycin) are shown in Table 11.1).

Mode of action of antimicrobial agents

There are five main modes of action of antibiotics:

(1) *Inhibition of cell-wall synthesis*. This involves inhibition of the transpeptidase step required for cross-linking the polysaccharide chains in the peptidoglycan layer of the cell wall. The penicillins, cephalosporins and cycloserine act in this way.

(2) *Damage to cell membrane*. Damage by binding to the membrane results in the loss of the semipermeable properties of the membrane. Substances then pass out from the cell and death occurs. Polypeptide antibiotics such as polymyxin and amphotericin act in this fashion.

(3) *Inhibition of protein synthesis*. Antibiotics causing this have an effect on translation in the cell and include chloramphenicol, the tetractclines, the amnioglycosides, erythromycin, lincomycin and clindamycin.

(4) *Inhibition of nucleic acid synthesis*. Nalidixic acid inhibits replication of DNA and rifampicin blocks transcription in prokaryotic cells.

(5) *Inhibition of folate synthesis*. Sulphonamides and trimethoprim block different steps in folate synthesis in bacteria.

Antibiotic resistance

Bacteria may be naturally resistant or, more commonly, may acquire resistance to drugs. Natural or innate resistance is exemplified by the resistance of *Escherichia coli* and some strains of *Staphylococcus aureus* to penicillin.

Acquired resistance, whereby bacteria initially sensitive to an antibiotic may become resistant, is produced by two mechanisms, mutation and gene transfer.

Mutation

Mutations develop spontaneously in bacterial cultures at a frequency of about one per 10^7 cell divisions, whether or not a drug has been administered. The resistant mutants that occur in the presence of antibiotic are not as robust as the parent strains and do not survive for long if the drug is discontinued. If, however, there is continued exposure to the antibiotic, sensitive parent strains will be killed whereas the resistant mutants will remain viable and multiply. The action of the drug therefore is to select the resistant bacteria (Fig. 11.1).

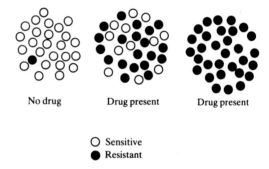

| No drug | Drug present | Drug present |

○ Sensitive
● Resistant

FIG. 11.1. Representation of the action of an antibiotic in selecting drug-resistant mutants.

The mechanism of resistance depends on the mode of action of the drug. For example, mutations may:

(1) produce decreased affinity of the site of action of the drug.

(2) reduce penetration of the drug into the cell by alteration of the cell membrane.

(3) cause inactivation of the drug by enzymes produced by the bacterium.

Gene transfer

This can occur by transduction or conjugation and consists of transfer of genetic material from a strain or species previously resistant to one or more antibiotic to a strain previously sensitive. In these cases genes for drug resistance are carried on extrachromosomal elements or plasmids.

Transduction. Penicillin resistance in *Staphylococcus aureus* depends on the presence of a plasmid carrying the gene for penicillinase (beta-lactamase) production. These plasmids can be transferred amongst different staphylococcal strains by bacteriophages.

Conjugation. R-factors are plasmids that bear drug-resistance genes and these may be spread by conjugation amongst cells of a wide range of Gram-negative species, notably the enterobacteria and *Pseudomonas aeruginosa.* Contact between donor and recipient cells is required and the genetic material is transferred directly between the two cells. This is a common form of resistance and is on the increase because of the widespread, and frequently unwise, use of antibiotics.

Transposons. Resistance determinants on *transposons,* which are transposable parts of nucleic acids can pass from plasmids to bacterial chromosomes or to phages and can be exchanged between plasmids. This explains how some forms of resistance can spread so quickly, and in a totally different way from recognised mechanisms.

Selection

Selection by antibiotics is important whether resistance is produced by mutation or by gene transfer. Repeated exposure of bacteria to the drug together with long periods of exposure in the population means that more resistant strains will be selected out. An important step in limiting the increasing number of resistant strains is to reduce or discontinue the use of the drug. This should allow the return of the sensitive strains. This is an important principle in the eradication of resistant strains in individuals and in the hospital environment where multiply-resistant strains have become established.

LABORATORY CONTROL OF ANTIMICROBIAL THERAPY

Such tests include assays on the organism as well as measurements of antibiotic levels in the patient.

Tests on the organism

These are of two types, disk sensitivity tests and dilution tests.

Disk diffusion tests. These are the tests most commonly used because they are rapid and convenient. Paper disks are impregnated with an antibiotic solution of known concentration (usually commerically obtained) and placed on the surface of an agar plate which has been inoculated with the test organism or the clinical specimen. After culture zones of inhibition of growth of the organism are examined and compared with a control organism. Provided conditions are standardised the degree of inhibition of growth round the disk gives some indication of the sensitivity of the organism (Fig. 11.2). Disk diffusion tests are not totally accurate and

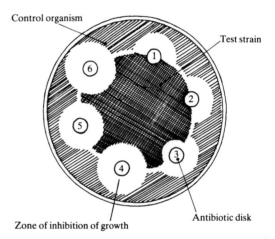

FIG. 11.2. Disk sensitivity test (Stokes' method). The test strain is resistant to antibiotics 1 and 2 moderately sensitive to antibiotic 3 and is sensitive to antibiotics 4, 5 and 6.

reliable because of the problems of inoculum size, composition of the medium, antibiotic content of the disk, pH and speed of growth of the test organism. It is possible to measure zone sizes and read the sensitivity or resistance for that antibiotic and strain from a pre-prepared regression-line graph. This method (Kirby–Bauer) is widely used in the U.S.A.

Dilution tests. These are of two types, tube dilution and agar plate dilution.

Tube dilution tests. These methods are too time-consuming and laborious for routine use but they are performed from time to time in all laboratories. They indicate the minimum inhibitory concentration (MIC) of a drug required for a specific organism in diseases such as infective endocarditis, thereby ensuring a more accurate and effective dose regimen. The MIC is read from the tube containing the highest dilution of the antibiotic that inhibits growth.

Agar plate dilution tests. These are useful when a large number of strains have to be tested. Various dilutions of the antibiotic are prepared in agar plates and each plate is seeded with several strains. After incubation the minimum bactericidal concentration (MBC) of the drug can be readily ascertained from the plate that contains the highest dilution of the antibiotic required to prevent growth of the test strain.

The MBC is determined by subculturing MIC tubes that show no growth on to solid media. The MBC is not necessarily the same as the MIC. It is more sensitive than the MIC in that it indicates the presence of small numbers of surviving or persisting bacteria. The phenomenon of persistence of organisms at antibiotic concentrations above the MIC is common.

Measurement of antibiotic levels in the patient

Assays can be performed on serum, urine, sputum or cerebrospinal fluid and these measure whether or not effective concentrations of an antibiotic are being attained. They are also useful in guarding against excessively high serum levels of antibiotics which may cause serious side effects. Tube dilution and agar diffusion methods may be used. In tube dilutions, graded dilutions of the fluid to be tested, usually serum, are made in a liquid medium; a standard inoculum of bacteria of known sensitivity, for example *Staphylococcus aureus* NCTC 6571, the Oxford staphylococcus, is then added. After incubation the tubes are examined for turbidity and the tube that contains the highest dilution of serum to inhibit growth of the organisms is noted. The MIC of the Oxford staphylococcus is known for each antibiotic and this allows calculation of the amount of antibiotic present in the patient's undiluted serum. It can also be helpful to check the patient's serum levels of antibiotic against the organism isolated as in the management of infective endocarditis.

Agar diffusion methods. Holes are cut in the agar previously inoculated with a control organism. The holes are filled with the serum under test and zones of inhibition produced by the antibiotic in the serum are compared with a graph of the sizes of zones produced by known concentrations of the antibiotic.

In guarding against excessive serum levels of a potentially toxic antibiotic such as gentamicin,

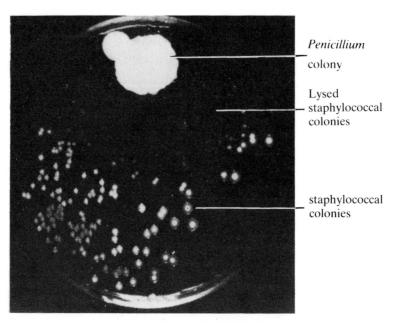

Penicillium colony

Lysed staphylococcal colonies

staphylococcal colonies

Fig. 11.3. The original observation of Fleming of the inhibition of growth of staphylococci by the mould *Penicillium*. From the *British Journal of Experimental Pathology* (1929) **10**, 228.

estimations can be made by testing serum taken about one hour after a dose (peak level) and serum taken just before the next dose (trough level). Many rapid and often semi-automated methods of detecting the aminoglycoside concentrations of serum samples are now available.

Antimicrobial drugs of clinical importance

The penicillins

In 1929 Sir Alexander Fleming discovered the antibiotic penicillin. He noted that a mould contaminant (*Penicillium notatum*) caused lysis of colonies of staphylococci growing in its immediate vicinity on a Petri dish (Fig. 11.3).

Mode of action. All are bactericidal, acting by inhibiting the glycopeptide transpeptidase required for cross-linking the peptide chains attached to the peptidoglycan layer of the cell wall. Because the transpeptidation step is completely blocked bacteria sensitive to penicillin become lysed during growth by osmosis, due to lack of a cell wall.

Resistance. This is common. Many strains of *Staphylococcus aureus* are now resistant because of the production of a penicillin-destroying enzyme, beta-lactamase, that hydrolyses the beta-lactam ring in the penicillin nucleus; such strains are common in hospital and are spread by cross infection. *Streptococcus faecalis* is naturally resistant to penicillin and *Haemophilus influenzae* is always at least moderately resistant. Many Gram-negative bacilli produce beta-lactamases. There is increasing resistance to penicillin in gonococci due either to mutation or the production of a beta-lactamase. Penicillins are virtually non-toxic although hypersensivity is a problem in some patients.

Antibacterial spectrum. This depends on the penicillin; the particular type of side-chain derivative largely determines the individual spectrum.

Table 11.2 shows the principal penicillins, their antibacterial spectrum and main indications for use.

The cephalosporins

Mode of action. All are bactericidal, beta-lactam antibiotics with a mode of action similar to penicillin.

Resistance. Many are resistant to beta-lactamases.

Antibacterial spectrum and uses. Three generations of cephalosporins have now been produced with different antibacterial effects and methods of administration. They can be given to patients who are hypersensitive to penicillin, although in a minority of cases cross-hypersensitivity occurs. There are now so

TABLE 11.2. The penicillins.

Type	Antibacterial spectrum	Uses
Benzyl penicillin (Penicillin G) (parenteral) Phenoxymethyl penicillin (Penicillin V) (oral)	Many gram-positive cocci and bacilli and Gram-negative cocci; spirochaetes	Infections caused by some staphylococci, beta-haemolytic streptococci; some viridans streptococci; pneumococci; clostridia, (tetanus, gas gangrene); anthrax; actinomycosis; syphilis; some cases of meningitis and gonorrhoea
Cloxacillin Flucloxacillin	Similar spectrum to penicillin G and V but less active. Resistant to staphylococcal beta-lactamase (penicillinase)	Staphylococcal infections
Ampicillin Amoxycillin	'Broad spectrum', i.e. same as penicillin G and V but, in addition, effective against most *Haemophilus influenzae*, *Streptococcus faecalis* and coliforms	Many respiratory, urinary tract and enteric infections.
Carbenicillin Ticarcillin	As ampicillin, but with activity against some strains of *Pseudomonas* and *Proteus* species	Respiratory and urinary tract infections and infections caused by *Pseudomonas*
Azlocillin Mezlocillin	Coliform organisms, particularly *Pseudomonas aeruginosa*	*Pseudomonas* infections
(Piv) mecillinam	Coliform organisms	Urinary tract infections

TABLE 11.3.   Some of the main cephalosporins.

Type	Antibacterial spectrum and uses

FIRST GENERATION
  Cephaloridine
  Cephalothin
  Cephalexin
	Many Gram-positive and Gram-negative organisms, although *Bacteroides* spp, *Pseudomonas* and *Haemophilus influenzae* are amongst the resistant bacteria. Sensitivity tests are mandatory.

SECOND GENERATION
  Cephamandole
  Cefoxitin
  (a cephamycin)
  Cefuroxime
	Improvements on first generation drugs, because of (1) greater stability to beta-lactamases and (2) activity against some of the bacteria (e.g. *Bacteroides*) resistant to first generation cephalosporins. Useful when aminoglycoside toxicity is a problem.

THIRD GENERATION Cefotaxime	Spectrum same as with second generation drugs with, in addition, activity against *Pseudomonas*. Less active against staphylococci.

many cephalosporin drugs on the commercial market that the choice of any particular drug is difficult and bewildering. There are, however, some that can be recommended for various infections and a selection of these with their uses is shown in Table 11.3.

Erythromycin

This is a macrolide antibiotic that is widely used against Gram-positive organisms such as beta-haemolytic streptococci, pneumococci and some *Staphylococcus aureus*, Gram-negative anaerobes and clostridia. It is not effective against the enterobacteria and most other Gram-negative bacilli although it is active against neisseriae, *Haemophilus influenzae*, *Bordetella pertussis*, *Campylobacter* spp, *Legionella* and some strains of *Bacteroides;* it has also an effect against chlamydiae and rickettsiae. It is particularly useful in the treatment of patients who are hypersensitive to penicillin.

Mode of action. Mainly bacteriostatic, though high doses may be bactericidal, it acts on bacterial ribosomes to inhibit protein synthesis.

Resistance. This arises rather easily by mutation in *Staphylococcus aureus*, streptococci and pneumococci, though resistant strains usually disappear if the drug is discontinued for a period.

The lincomycins

The two available drugs, clindamycin and lincomycin, are unrelated chemically to any other antibiotic. They are similar in many ways to erythromycin in antibacterial effects, mode of action and resistance. Cross resistance occurs amongst these drugs. Clindamycin is the newer, better absorbed and more active drug and has a greater effect against anaerobes. Both are useful in the treatment of infections caused by Gram-positive aerobes, such as *Staphylococcus aureus*, and because of very good penetration and diffusion in tissues such as bone they are recommended for the treatment of acute and chronic osteomyelitis. However, reports that these drugs can be associated with pseudo-membranous colitis may make the use of some other suitable drug more desirable.

Aminoglycosides

The following are included in this large group of antibiotics: streptomycin, kanamycin, amikacin, gentamicin, tobramycin, neomycin, netilmicin, framycetin.

Mode of action. These are bactericidal drugs and act on bacterial ribosomes to produce inhibition of protein synthesis by interfering with messenger RNA attachment. As absorption from the gut is minimal administration is either topical (neomycin, framycetin) or parenteral (other aminoglycosides).

Resistance. This is caused by the acquisition of enzymes by the bacteria that can denature the drug. Gentamicin is the most useful drug in the group, with activity against many coliforms, and particularly against *Pseudomonas aeruginosa*. Tobramycin and amikacin may be used in cases of gentamicin resistance.

Tetracyclines

These include tetracycline, chlortetracycline, oxytetracycline, doxycycline, minocycline, dimethyl-chlortetracycline.

Mode of action. These drugs are bacteriostatic, inhibiting protein synthesis by preventing the attachment of amino acids to ribosomes.

Resistance. Usually plasmid-mediated this is now becoming common.

Antibacterial spectrum and uses. The spectrum of antibacterial effect is broad and many Gram-positive and Gram-negative bacteria can be affected, as well as *Mycoplasma pneumoniae, Coxiella burneti* and chlamydiae. The drugs are particularly useful in the prophylaxis and treatment of acute and chronic bronchitis, non-specific urethritis, atypical pneumonia and Q fever.

Chloramphenicol

Antibacterial spectrum and uses. A broad-spectrum antibiotic, chloramphenicol is effective against most pathogenic bacteria, with the exception of *Pseudomonas* spp, but because of its toxic side effects on the bone marrow and its possible role in causing circulatory collapse in infants its use must be severely limited to certain infections, notably *Haemophilus influenzae* meningitis in children and the acute stages of typhoid fever; for both of these infections it is the drug of choice. It can be used locally in the eye for conjunctivitis.

Mode of action. Chloramphenicol produces its bacteriostatic effect by inhibiting protein synthesis.

Resistance. Resistance to chloramphenicol is present on the R-factors of many coliform bacilli particularly in countries where it is still widely available without prescription.

Sulphonamides

Sulphadiazine and sulphadimidine are widely used drugs.

Mode of action. Sulphonamides are structural analogues of paraaminobenzoic acid (PABA) which is involved in the synthesis of folic acid by bacteria. They inhibit bacterial growth by competitive inhibition of the enzymes involved in the incorporation of PABA into the folate pathway.

Resistance. Many species, particularly meningococci, in the past sensitive to the sulphonamides, are now resistant and this applies also to other bacteria. Resistance can be produced by synthesis of a folic

acid synthetase that has a lowered affinity for sulphonamide, or by over-production of PABA. Cross resistance in the group is complete.

Antibacterial spectrum and uses. These drugs have a broad-spectrum, bacteriostatic effect. They are effective against certain Gram-positive organisms such as pneumococci but their use against these organisms has been superseded by other drugs. Some Gram-negative cocci are sensitive and also many enterobacteria. Sulphonamides are used against Gram-negative bacilli, for example in urinary tract infection caused by *Escherichia coli* and certain non-absorbable varieties can be used for preoperative preparation of the bowel.

Sulphonamides and trimethoprim

Cotrimoxazole is a bacteriostatic combination of sulphamethoxazole and trimethoprim in a 5:1 ratio.

Mode of action. Trimethoprim is a synthetic agent that in concert with sulphonamides produces a sequential blockade of folic acid synthesis in bacteria which results *in vitro* in a synergistic action.

Resistance. This can be produced by production of enzymes in bacteria that are resistant to both drugs.

Antibacterial spectrum and uses. As a broad-spectrum combination it is effective against many Gram-positive and Gram-negative bacteria. It is very effective against *Haemophilus influenzae* and therefore widely used for acute and chronic bronchitis and against many of the organisms that cause urinary tract infections.

Trimethoprim

This drug is now available on its own and can be used for respiratory and urinary tract infections. It has fewer side effects than cotrimoxazole.

Fusidic acid

Mode of action. Fusidic acid inhibits protein synthesis and is bacteriostatic.

Resistance. Resistance to the drug is plasmid-borne.

Antibacterial spectrum and uses. Fusidic acid is effective against many Gram-positive cocci, Gram-negative cocci and Gram-positive bacilli but its outstanding action is against *Staphylococcus aureus*. It has been used successfully in acute and chronic forms of staphylococcal disease such as osteomyelitis, deep sepsis and septicaemia. It should be used in combination with other antistaphylococcal drugs to reduce the likelihood of resistance to this bacteriostatic agent.

Nalidixic acid

Mode of action. DNA replication is inhibited.

Antibacterial spectrum and uses. This drug is active against many coliform organisms (excluding *Pseudomonas aeruginosa)* and is used in the treatment of urinary tract infections.

Nitrofurantoin

Active against coliform organisms (not *Pseudomonas aeruginosa*) and *Streptococcus faecalis*, it is useful for urinary tract infections because of its rapid excretion into the urine.

The polypeptides

Antibacterial spectrum and uses. These antibiotics are nearly all too toxic for systemic use but can be of value as topical agents in infections of the eye, ear and burns. Colistin (polymyxin E), the only member that can be given systemically, is active against *Pseudomonas aeruginosa.*

Rifamycins

In combination with other antituberculous drugs rifampicin can be used successfully in the treatment of tuberculosis. A combination with another drug is desirable because resistance develops rapidly.

Vancomycin

This bactericidal drug is effective against Gram-positive bacteria and can be used in cases of septicaemia and infective endocarditis. It is a useful reserve antibiotic and it should therefore not be used routinely.

Metronidazole

This compound belongs to the nitroimidazole group and for many years was used to treat infections with the protozoon *Trichomonas vaginalis* and other protozoon infections. Acute ulceromembranous gingivitis (Vincent's gingivitis) was also known to respond more rapidly to metronidazole than to penicillin. Some years after metronidazole was introduced to treat these two infections its wider role as an agent capable of killing anaerobic bacteria was realised. Since about 1978 use of this antibiotic has increased dramatically and it is firmly established in Europe as the agent of choice in anaerobic infections. It is also used as a prophylactic agent where anaerobic infections are possible sequelae of surgery.

Mode of action. Metronidazole has a disputed mode of action but it seems to depend on reduction of the nitro group of the molecule, which in turn acts on the DNA of the bacterium or protozoon. The drug is itself inactivated in the process of killing the organism.

Resistance. Resistance to metronidazole is virtually unknown amongst strict anaerobes. Indeed, sensitivity to metronidazole is often used by laboratories as a quick check that an organism is a strict anaerobe. Microaerophilic bacteria or capnophilic bacteria such as microaerophilic Gram-positive cocci, *Eikenella corrodens*, *Campylobacter sputorum* and *Capnocytophaga ochracea* are therefore resistant.

TABLE 11.4.   Organisms sensitive to metronidazole.

Trichomonas vaginalis
Bacteroides
Fusobacterium
Leptotrichia buccalis
Veillonella
Clostridium spp
Anaerobic cocci

Antimicrobial spectrum and uses. The drug should not be used in the first trimester of pregnancy and patients taking it should refrain from alcohol whilst the therapy continues. Anaerobic infections may be treated orally, parenterally or with suppositories or pessaries. The spectrum of organisms sensitive to metronidazole is given in Table 11.4.

Antifungal drugs

Nystatin

Mode of action. Nystatin is a polyene anti-fungal agent with activity restricted to the yeast-like fungi such as a *Candida* spp. It acts by combining with sterols in the yeast cell membrane and increases permeability of the membrane to cell contents. These leak out causing death of the yeast.

Spectrum and uses. It is used topically as cream or ointment on mucosae or skin infected with candida. Tablets can be sucked or swallowed to treat oral and gastro-intestinal candidosis. Pessaries are available for vaginal infections. Fortunately, because of poor absorption, nystatin has little systemic effect as the drug is toxic for mammalian cells.

Nystatin is much used for oral and peri-oral candidal infections. It is usually given in tablet form but there is also ointment and cream. The ointment is smeared on the commissures in angular cheilitis and the cream is smeared on the fitting surface of dentures as an adjunct to therapy for denture stomatitis.

Resistance. Unknown among yeast-like fungi.

Amphotericin

Spectrum and uses. This similar polyene anti-fungal agent has potent activity against filamentous fungi such as *Aspergillus fumigatus* as well as the yeast-like fungi. It is toxic even in small doses if administered systemically but for many years it was the only suitable agent for systemic mycotic infections.

Oral infections are treated with lozenges; these are allowed to dissolve in the mouth, their taste being more pleasant than nystatin. Cream and ointment are available and are used as described for nystatin.

Mode of action. Similar to nystatin.

Resistance. None among yeast like fungi.

Miconazole

Spectrum and uses. This is a member of the imidazole group of anti-fungal agents, drugs active against all pathogenic fungi including dermatophytes, filamentous and dimorphic fungi and yeasts. Miconazole can be administered topically or parenterally and is well absorbed from the gastrointestinal tract. It is fairly well tolerated and safe. It is administered for oral infections as an oral gel or in tablet form; the gel can be allowed to dissolve in the mouth before swallowing. There is no suitable vehicle yet available for application of miconazole to dentures or to commissures. Two other imidazoles, ketaconazole and clot-

rimazole can be administered topically for oral infections with the yeast-like fungi but further evaluation of these is required.

Flucytosine (5-fluorocytosine)

This drug is used for systemic yeast infections and is safer than amphotericin with which it is sometimes combined. Griseofulvin is used to treat dermatophyte infections and is not effective against the yeast-like fungi. It is not used in the mouth.

Treatment of oral yeast infections.

Although many oral infections with *Candida albicans* and related yeast-like fungi respond quickly to drug therapy some infections persist stubbornly. Often predisposing factors such as wearing dentures at night and systemic disease, drugs or debilitation are the cause of this. It would appear that none of these infections is caused by resistant strains of yeasts and a careful elimination of predisposing factors to infection is often the only course open to the clinician. The systemic and topical action of miconazole may be helpful in some of these cases but a full evaluation has yet to be made. Table 11.5 shows the length of time of treatment with anticandidal drugs (amphotericin or nystatin) required to achieve a resolution of infection in patients attending the Oral Medicine Clinic in the Manchester Dental Hospital in 1977.

Antiviral agents

Idoxuridine

At the present time this is the most frequently used antiviral agent for oral and peri-oral infections. It is

TABLE 11.5. Length of treatment with anticandidal drugs.

Time	Cases with clinical cure	
	No.	%
2 weeks	26	27.4
1 month	27	28.4
2 months	19	20.0
3 months	7	7.3
6 months	4	4.2
1 year	5	5.3
>1 year	7	7.4
Total	95	

active against DNA viruses in which it inhibits the incorporation of thymidine into the DNA of replicating viral genomes. Despite the potential danger of similar changes occurring in host DNA idoxuridine has a good record of safety when used topically on skin and on the eye, although it is now regarded as too toxic for systemic use. If necessary oral (usually primary) and peri-oral (usually recurrent) infections with herpes simplex virus may be treated with 0.1 per cent idoxuridine paint, in purified water. This is also the preparation used for herpetic eye infections. Herpetic skin infections such as zoster can be treated with 5 per cent idoxuridine in dimethylsulphoxide. Both preparations should be applied to early lesions up to five times daily to have any prospect of benefit.

Cytarabine

This agent again acts against viral DNA and has been used systemically in severe infections with herpes viruses, usually in compromised patients such as those with leukaemia.

Vidarabine

Similar to cytarabine this agent is less toxic for human cells. It has been used with some success for systemic herpes virus infections, herpetic eye infections, cytomegalovirus infections and hepatitis B infection.

Acyclovir

This new drug has shown considerable promise as an antiviral agent for herpetic ulceration of the cornea and for systemic and genital infections with herpes virus. Toxicity appears to be low. The agent acts by inhibiting the viral DNA polymerase much more actively than that of the host cells.

Interferon

Interferons are naturally occurring substances produced by host cells in response to viral infection that afford some protection against further cell infection by the virus. Interferon molecules are generally species-specific but modern biotechnological methods have enabled therapeutic amounts of 'human' interferon to be produced. Interferon has been shown to be effective to varying degrees in herpetic keratitis, herpes zoster infections, influenza and hepatitis B infections. This activity against viruses has been largely overshadowed by the potential use of interferon as a therapeutic agent for certain neoplastic diseases.

FURTHER READING

Garrod L.P., Lambert H.P. & O'Grady F. (1981) *Antibiotic and Chemotherapy*, 5th Edition. Edinburgh: Churchill Livingstone.

Ball A.P., Gray J.A. & Murdoch J. McC. (1978) *Antibacterial Drugs Today*, 2nd Edition. Lancaster: MTP Press.

Dental Practitioners' Formulary (1982) London: British Medical Association, and The Pharmaceutical Press.

Ross P.W. (1983) *Journal of Maternal and Child Health*, **8**, 110–116.

CHAPTER 12

The Ecology of the Mouth

The mouth harbours many microorganisms in an ecosystem of considerable complexity that has not been fully investigated yet and is far from completely understood. Until quite recently the mouth was regarded as a single habitat for microorganisms but it is now realised that the teeth, gingival crevice, tongue, other mucosal surfaces and saliva all form different habitats or sites where microorganisms multiply. Each habitat contains its own characteristic population often with many different microbial species. These species may complement or compete with others in the same population and thus the oral flora is a dynamic entity affected by many changes throughout the life of the host.

DEVELOPMENT OF THE ORAL FLORA

Birth

The mouth of the full-term foetus is usually sterile, although organisms which are only transient may be acquired from the vagina at birth. The mouth of the newborn baby rapidly acquires organisms from the mother and also from the environment. Several streptococcal and staphylococcal species may be isolated, together with coliforms, lactobacilli, *Bacillus* spp, *Neisseria* spp and yeasts. The selectivity of the mouth as an environment is demonstrated even at this time because most of the organisms introduced fail to become established. *Streptococcus salivarius* is the most common isolate from the mouths of young babies and together with *Staphylococcus albus, Neisseria* spp and *Veillonella* spp they form the pioneer community. Occasionally *Candida albicans* multiplies rapidly in the mouth and the low pH it produces prevents the normal growth of other commensals. A florid overgrowth of yeasts produces what is known as 'oral thrush'.

Infancy and early childhood

The infant comes into contact with an ever-increasing range of microorganisms and some of these will become established as part of the commensal flora of the individual. Commensal organisms in other sites of the body and organisms from the environment will be presented to the oral cavity and some will become established. The eruption of deciduous teeth provides a different surface for microbial attachment and this is characterised by the appearance of *Streptococcus sanguis* and *mutans* as regular inhabitants of the oral cavity. With increasing numbers of teeth and changes in diet the overall proportions of organisms in the mouth will change. A few anaerobes become established but as there is no deep gingival crevice the numbers remain small. Actinomycetes, lactobacilli and *Rothia* are found regularly.

Adolescence

Perhaps the greatest increase in numbers of organisms in the mouth occurs when the permanent teeth erupt. These teeth have deep fissures in their surfaces that do not readily wear down. The interproximal spaces are much larger than in the deciduous dentition as the teeth have a more pronounced 'neck' at the amelo-cemental junction. The gingival crevice is deeper than in the deciduous dentition and allows for a great increase in anaerobic organisms. *Bacteroides* spp become established in large numbers as well as *Leptotrichia* spp, *Fusobacterium* spp and spirochaetes. The lesions of

71

dental caries will create a new environment in which some organisms especially streptococci will flourish. In ecological terms the oral flora of late adolescence and early adulthood, before the loss of teeth, is the climax community.

Adulthood

The complexity of the oral flora of the adult is perhaps its chief characteristic. Varying amounts of dental plaque may be present and the degree of chronic periodontal disease will also govern the numbers and types of microorgansims found. Carious lesions and unsatisfactory restorations will provide environments for local accumulations of bacteria. Most studies of the adult oral flora show that considerable variation occurs among individuals in total numbers and proportions of many species of bacteria; indeed there may be variation within one individual when sampled on several occasions.

Consistent with the trends seen in adolescence there is an increase in the *Bacteroides* spp and spirochaetes with advancing periodontal disease and maturity of dental plaque. Superficial plaque contains many streptococci, mostly *Streptococcus mutans*, *mitior (mitis)* and *sanguis*. Actinomycetes and other Gram-positive and Gram-negative filaments of uncertain taxonomic position are also regularly isolated.

As teeth are lost so the numbers of available sites for microbial colonisation decrease; the numbers of bacteria decrease and several species diminish disproportionately in numbers. Edentulous patients harbour few spirochaetes or bacteroides but their carriage of yeasts increases. Yeasts are normally found on the dorsum of the tongue and in the upper buccal sulcus. Dentures provide a protected environment in which yeasts can multiply, covering the hard palate and the acrylic denture surface.

Factors affecting the development of the oral flora

In order to become established in the mouth an organism must (1) be introduced, (2) be retained and (3) be able to multiply in the conditions present in the mouth.

(1) Introduction

Although from birth a wide variety of microorganisms are introduced into the mouth only certain species are able to become established in the oral cavity. Many of these organisms have a predilection for particular sites such as lips, dorsum of tongue, hard palate, other soft tissues, gingival crevice or teeth.

(2) Retention

Retention of microorganisms is usually confined to a particular site in the mouth, presumably as a result of the often complex interplay of detaching and retentive factors.

Adherence: Some bacteria have the ability to adhere to soft tissues; *Streptococcus salivarius* can adhere to the mucosa of the dorsum of the tongue and also to other soft tissues. Others, in particular *Streptococcus mutans*, *mitior* and *sanguis* adhere to enamel as the result of the production of extracellular polysaccharide. It is likely that some oral actinomycetes adhere through a hyaluronic acid-mediated mechanism. Other bacteria may merely stick to the extra-cellular matrix produced by others. Weakly-adhering bacteria such as *Veillonella* spp will also lodge in enamel defects, occlusal fissures and pits where they are protected from dislodging forces.

Protected sites: In addition to the above the sticky matrix of dental plaque will provide a protected environment for those bacteria which do not possess any adherence mechanisms. However, the largest protected site is the gingival crevice where species such as *Bacteroides melaninogenicus* and spirochaetes can survive.

Detachment forces: These include salivary flow, the movement of tongue and soft tissues and the abrasive action of the diet. The flow of gingival crevice fluid and phagocytosis in the crevice also serve to remove bacteria.

(3) Multiplication

To become established as a member of the oral flora an organism must be able to multiply in the particular site in which it can be retained. A number of factors govern this.

Availability of substrates: In order to grow bacteria must be able to metabolise the available substrates which come in the diet or in the metabolic products of other organisms in the same or a related site. Increased carbohydrate in the diet probably has the greatest effects in increasing the numbers of oral bacteria, especially streptococci.

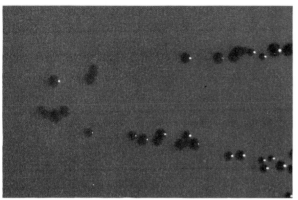

PLATE 1. *Bacteroides melaninogenicus* on blood agar to show black-pigmented colonies.

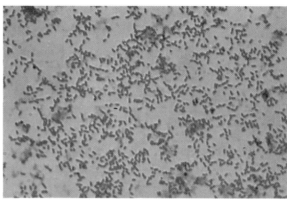

PLATE 2. Gram stain of *Bacteroides melaninogenicus* showing Gram-negative pleomorphic rods.

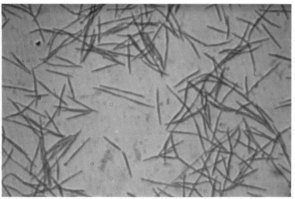

PLATE 3. Gram stain of *Fusobacterium nucleatum* showing Gram-negative rods with pointed ends.

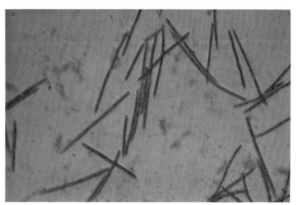

PLATE 4. Gram stain of *Leptotrichia buccalis* showing large Gram-negative rods.

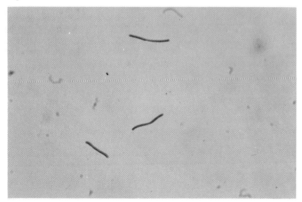

PLATE 5. Gram stain of *Bacterionema matruchotii* showing a short Gram-positive rod with a long Gram-positive filament protruding from it.

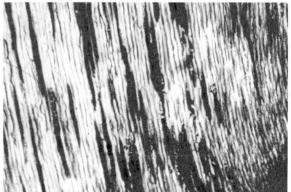

PLATE 6. Bacteria in dentinal tubules viewed in longitudinal section. Courtesy of Professor J. C. Southam.

pH: The metabolism of microorganisms is often dependent on pH and bacteria inhibited by low pH may not survive in the acid conditions of dental plaque or under the base of a denture. *Bacteroides melaninogenicus* and *Veillonella* spp are intolerant of pH below about 5.5 but *Lactobacillus* spp and *Candida albicans* can tolerate very low pH values.

Oxidation or reduction of surroundings: The oxidation-reduction potential (Eh) of the site is often crucial in determining the nature of the flora in that site. Anaerobic organisms such as bacteroides, fusobacteria, spirochaetes and some actinomycetes will only multiply in reduced surroundings. The requirements for reduction are varied; actinomycetes, *Capnocytophaga* spp and *Campylobacter* spp require a less reduced environment than *Bacteroids* spp, fusobacteria and particularly spirochaetes. Low oxidation-reduction potential can only be achieved readily in the gingival crevice and in the deeper layer of dental plaque. This goes some way to explaining why these anaerobic bacteria are confined to such sites.

Microbial interactions: The complexity of communities of microorganisms is the result of a number of microbial interactions. Some of these are nutritional such as the provision of para-amino benzoic acid by *Streptococcus sanguis* for *Streptococcus mutans* in reduced conditions; the provision of vitamin K by several microorganisms for *Bacteroides melaninogenicus* which in turn produces formate for *Campylobacter sputorum*. Spirochaetes are dependent on a number of factors produced by several bacteria, perhaps indicating why these organisms can only become established in the gingival crevices after the remainder of the normal flora has developed.

Some interactions are detrimental rather than beneficial to a second species; for example the production of hydrogen peroxide by *Streptococcus sanguis* inhibits many other streptococci and anaerobes. Inhibitory substances termed bacteriocins that act on different strains of the same or related species have been noted among oral streptococci and *Bacteroides* spp. The inhibition of a microorganism by another may well produce an adjacent vacant site that can then be colonised by the first microorganism to multiply.

The competition to occupy all the available sites in the mouth gives rise to the dynamic nature of the normal flora but it is also of benefit to the host in helping to prevent the establishment in the mouth of any pathogen that may be introduced.

THE NORMAL MICROBIAL FLORA OF DIFFERENT SITES OF THE MOUTH

Lips

On the lips there is a transition from skin to oral mucosa and there are also changes in the bacterial population. *Staphylococcus albus* and skin micrococci predominate with large numbers of streptococci typical of the mouth. If the commissures are moistened by saliva an angular cheilitis may develop from which *Candida albicans*, *Staphylococcus aureus* and *Streptococcus pyogenes* may be cultured.

Cheek

The results of studies vary to some degree but the predominant cheek bacterium is *Streptococcus mitior* with *Streptococcus sanguis* and *salivarius* the next most common. Yeasts may be isolated from carriers and other organisms present in saliva will be washed over the surface of the cheek and may be retained for some time, for example *Haemophilus* and *Neisseria* spp.

Palate

The hard palate supports a streptococcal flora resembling the cheek. Haemophili are found regularly and lactobacilli are common. The few anaerobes found on exposed mucosal surfaces almost certainly do not multiply. Yeasts and lactobacilli will increase dramatically in some denture wearers and the flora may alter substantially when the palate is protected from the action of tongue and saliva by a denture base. The soft palate will harbour respiratory tract bacteria such as *Haemophilus*, *Cornebacterium*, *Neisseria* and *Branhamella*. Carriers of beta-haemolytic streptococci will often have the organisms on the uvula, the palato-glossal and palato-pharyngeal folds.

Tongue

The keratinised dorsal surface of the tongue is an ideal site for the retention of microorganisms. Although the reported numbers vary *Streptococcus salivarius* is the predominant organism, representing 20–50 per cent of the total cultivable flora. *Streptococcus mitior* is also common and *Haemophilus* spp have been regularly isolated. The dorsum of the tongue is frequently colonised by small numbers of *Candida albicans*. *Micrococcus mucilagenous* is an unusual organism that resembles a staphylococcus but produces an extracellular slime

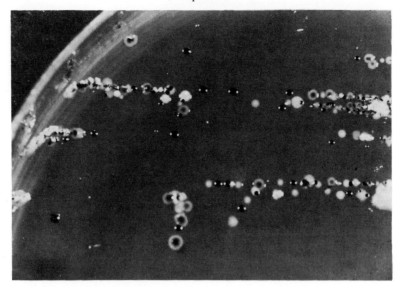

FIG. 12.1. Bacterial colonies isolated from the gingival crevice.

that may account for its retention on the tongue. The organism represents 3-4 per cent of the cultivable flora in most subjects and is isolated only from the dorsum of the tongue.

Gingival crevice

The bacterial population of the gingival crevice is perhaps the most numerous of any site in the mouth with 10^{10}–10^{11} organisms per gram wet weight of gingival debris (Fig. 12.1). There have been many studies of the gingival crevice and closely related to these studies on dental plaque, either supra- or sub-gingival. (A more detailed account of dental plaque is presented in Chap. 13). The gingival crevice is relatively well protected from the forces that dislodge bacteria and the crevicular fluid transudate provides a rich nutrient medium that enables some relatively fastidious organisms to thrive. Despite the proximity of oxygen in the air and blood the gingival crevice has a low Eh which may achieve levels of –300 m.V. in a deep periodontal pocket. Metabolism of substrates in the crevice by facultative organisms, microaerophils, and the less strict anaerobes contributes to a progressive lowering of the Eh so that spirochaetes can grow at values below –180 m.V.

The exact numbers and proportions of the various organisms present in the gingival crevice vary with different sampling and cultural techniques. Table 12.1 gives the mean values of four reports of well-conducted studies.

TABLE 12.1. The percentage cultivable flora from the gingival crevice area of man.

Facultative Gram-positive cocci	27.0
Anaerobic Gram-positive cocci	10.0
Facultative Gram-negative cocci	1.0
Anaerobic Gram-negative cocci	10.9
Facultative Gram-positive rods and filaments	13.5
Anaerobic Gram-positive rods and filaments	20.3
Facultative Gram-negative rods and filaments	0.9
Anaerobic Gram-negative rods and filaments	20.4
Spiral forms	2 **

** Spirochaetes estimated microscopically and not recorded in some studies.

Teeth

All erupted teeth have microorganisms attached usually in the deposits termed dental plaque. Forces that detach bacteria such as food, saliva and the soft tissues tend to remove dental plaque from the smooth enamel surface lingually or palatally and buccally. These bacterial deposits build up initially as follows:

(1) in the occlusal fissures and pits.
(2) in enamel defects.
(3) in interproximal spaces.
(4) close to the gingival margin.

The viable count of dental plaque may only represent a proportion of the total count. Variations in plaque composition are wide but oral streptococci, Gram-positive rods and filaments and some Gram-negative anaerobes are always present.

Saliva

The salivary flora was for many years regarded as representative of the oral flora as a whole but the increasing understanding of the differences in microbial populations of various anatomical sites in the oral cavity now makes this view untenable. The microbial count of saliva has been reported as between 10^7–10^8 organisms per ml. Most of these are washed out of their normal habitat and are swallowed after a short time, or succeed in being retained at another site in the mouth. Salivary counts of particular species of bacteria do not reflect the numbers at other sites in the mouth and this fact alone somewhat invalidates the various quantitative tests (such as lactobacillus counts) that were once used to assess susceptibility to dental caries.

Salivary samples can be useful in detecting carriers of *Candida albicans* or beta-haemolytic streptococci. Intended isolation of these organisms is probably the only indication nowadays for taking a salivary specimen for bacteriological examination although saliva may still be useful for the isolation of viruses.

Dentures and other intra-oral appliances

Any appliance worn in the mouth for a considerable period will itself become colonised with microorganisms and may alter the oral flora. Fixed orthodontic appliances often support considerable amounts of supra-gingival plaque and restorations, especially if poorly constructed, also harbour dental plaque. In general, foreign material placed permanently in the mouth is less well cleansed than are the natural oral tissues by the physiological self-cleansing mechanisms. Removable appliances have the advantage of being able to be cleansed properly and allowing a clearing of the stagnation areas in the mouth during the period of removal. If the appliance covers the palate there will be changes in the palatal flora but this may revert to normal during periods when the appliance is out of the mouth. Yeasts and lactobacilli in particular will multiply on any mucosal surface protected from the flow of saliva. Clasps and other parts of the appliance that cause stagnation will promote the build up of dental plaque. The appliance itself will absorb microorganisms on to its surface, a property that depends to a great extent on the material used. Acrylic appliances retain a denser flora than metal, probably because they are slightly porous and easily scratched, producing areas where microbes can be retained. Chemical bonding to acrylic may also occur. Few studies have been carried out into the microbial flora of appliances used in the mouth but it is known that yeasts, especially *Candida albicans* can be cultured in large numbers from the fitting surfaces of acrylic dentures.

THE PRINCIPAL MICROORGANISMS OF THE MOUTH

Some organisms described below are present in all mouths in large numbers, others are found in small numbers and some may be only transient in any one individual. Some are isolated regularly from only a proportion of a population. Unfortunately microbiological techniques are not yet sufficiently refined to yield quantitative data either about some fastidious organisms or those present in small numbers. It is salutary to realise that an organism present in dental plaque at a concentration of 10^3 per gram wet weight would only be encountered once in every 10–100 million cultivable microorganisms. Many microorganisms have been little studied and much remains to be confirmed about their characteristics and proportions in the normal oral flora. Not surprisingly many organisms have been re-classified as knowledge about them has increased and many new organisms have been discovered.

Gram-positive cocci

Streptococci

The oral streptococci comprise a group of bacteria that are either non-haemolytic or produce variable haemolytic patterns. For many years they were termed *Streptococcus viridans* but it has been realised for some time now that this group comprises at least five distinct species: *Streptococcus sanguis, mitior, mutans, salivarius* and *milleri*. These are now known as the 'viridans streptococci'. They dominate the oral flora in early life and in the climax community they represent about half the bacteria on the tongue, other mucosal surface and in saliva. They comprise about 30 per cent of the flora of dental plaque and the gingival crevice. Table 12.2 is a guide to the differentiation of these species.

Streptococcus sanguis is a common constituent of dental plaque because it adheres readily to the tooth surface through the production of extracellular glucan.

Streptococcus mitior is also a common constituent of dental plaque and some strains produce extracellular insoluble glucan while others do not. The glucan-producing strains resemble *Streptococcus sanguis* in many ways.

TABLE 12.2. Differentiation of species of oral streptococci.

| Species | Fermentation of | | Ammonia from arginine | Hydrolysis of aesculin | Acetoin production (V.P. test) | H_2O_2 production | Polysaccharide production from sucrose | |
	Mannitol	Sorbitol					Colonies (1)	Chemical nature
Streptococcus mutans	+	+	−	+	+	−	HARD	mutan
" *sanguis*	−	−	+	+	−	+	HARD	glucan
" *mitior*	−	−	−	−	+/−	+	HARD/SOFT[2]	glucan
" *milleri*	−	−	+	+	+	−	SOFT	−
" *salivarius*	−	−	−	+	−	−	MUCOID	fructan

+   majority of strains give a positive reaction.
−   majority of strains give a negative reaction.
+/− variable reaction.

(1)   On sucrose-containing agar plates.
(2)   Some strains produce hard colonies, some soft.

Courtesy of Dr. P. Marsh. *Oral Microbiology*. Van Nostrand Reinhold.

Streptococcus mutans is the bacterium widely regarded as causing the initial carious lesion on a tooth. Several serotypes are recognised (Bratthall serotypes a-g). Types c and d are most commonly implicated in dental caries particularly in Europe and North America. *Streptococcus mutans* produces a number of extracellular carbohydrate polymers from dietary sucrose including mutan and glucan. These polymers can attach firmly to the tooth and the bacteria attach to the polymers.

Streptococcus salivarius is mostly found attached to epithelial surfaces, particularly the dorsum of the tongue. It produces fructan from dietary sucrose. When grown on sucrose-containing agar the colonies are characteristically mucoid.

Streptococcus milleri is unusual among oral streptococci in that it does not produce any extracellular carbohydrate polymers. It does not show any particular preference for sites in the mouth although it is highly specific in the tissues in which it causes disease, such as the brain and liver.

Other aerobic streptococci isolated from the mouth include *Streptococcus faecalis* and *bovis*. A number of strictly anaerobic Gram-positive streptococci have been isolated regularly but the classification of these organisms is so uncertain that they are best described merely as anaerobic cocci at present. Some authorities place anaerobic cocci in the genus *Peptostreptococcus*. These strict anaerobes are isolated chiefly from the gingival crevice and the deeper areas of dental plaque.

Isolation of beta-haemolytic streptococci (Lancefield's groups A, B, C, F and G) is possible from the posterior soft palate and the tonsillar region in carriers.

Staphylococci

The lips harbour a number of staphylococci and micrococci but the intra-oral mucosal surfaces do not harbour many of these micro-organisms. This is in sharp contrast to the skin where staphylococci and micrococci predominate. *Micrococcus mucilagenous* is a regular isolate from the dorsum of the tongue but the incidence of other staphylococci and micrococci is somewhat unclear. No preferential site has been described for them in the mouth.

Gram-negative cocci

Neisseria and Branhamella

A number of Gram-negative diplococci are found in the mouth and these form part of the pioneer community. The oral strains of *Neisseria* include *Neisseria pharyngis* (synonyms: *flava, sicca*) and, among carriers, *Neisseria meningitidis* may be isolated from the throat. The remaining Gram-negative diplococci belong to the genus *Branhamella*, mostly *Branhamella catarrhalis*. These are isolated from dental plaque as well as from most mucosal surfaces, usually in small numbers.

Veillonella

This group of Gram-negative anaerobic cocci comprises two species *Veillonella parvula* and *alkalescens.* They are both found principally in dental plaque and are among the earliest anaerobes to colonise the mouth.

Gram-positive rods and filaments

There are numerous genera of Gram-positive rods and filaments represented in the mouth, mostly found in dental plaque. Isolation and characterisation of some of them may be quite difficult and the classification of these oral isolates is far from complete. Currently accepted genera are listed in Table 12.3.

TABLE 12.3. Gram-positive rods and filaments found in the mouth.

Genus	Atmosphere for growth
Lactobacillus	Aerobic/anaerobic
Corynebacterium	Aerobic
Bacillus	Aerobic
Actinomyces	Aerobic/anaerobic
Arachnia	Anaerobic
Eubacterium	Anaerobic
Propionibacterium	Anaerobic
Bacterionema	Aerobic
Rothia	Aerobic/microaerophilic
Bifidobacterium	Anaerobic
Clostridium	Anaerobic

Lactobacillus

These organisms appear as early colonisers of the mouth and remain as oral commensals, although in relatively small numbers. Two species are commonly found in the mouth, *Lactobacillus casei* and *acidophilus* although others can be isolated. Differentiation of the 27 recognised species of lactobacilli is often very difficult.

Corynebacterium

Members of this genus are found in almost all sites of the body where there is a commensal flora. They are often grouped together as 'diphtheroids' because of their similarity to *Corynebacterium diphtheriae.* Few oral corynebacteria can be assigned to a recognised species. These organisms are commensal and non-pathogenic. In the U.K. isolations of toxigenic and non-toxigenic *Corynebacterium diphtheriae* from the throat and soft palate occur from time to time.

Bacillus

These sporing Gram-positive rods are occasionally isolated from the mouth but are regarded as transient bacteria.

Actinomyces

A number of species of Gram-positive, usually branching, filaments of the genus *Actinomyces* have been isolated from the mouth. They are generally found in dental plaque but also inhabit the gingival crevice. The less anaerobic strains can multiply on mucosal surfaces as actinomycetes may be relatively early colonisers of the mouth. The oral species are mostly facultative anaerobes with only *Actinomyces israelii* regarded as a true anaerobe. This genus illustrates well the varying demands of bacteria for low Eh potentials for growth. *Actinomyces israelii* is a commensal and opportunistic pathogen but the other species are less pathogenic (Plates 11 and 12) *Actinomyces odontolyticus* was first isolated from carious dentine and it may be partly responsible for the progression of the lesion; *Actinomyces viscosus* and *naeslundii* are found in dental plaque and are closely related species that can be grouped together as a single species. *Actinomyces bovis* is not an oral commensal and as its name suggests has been found largely in the mouths of cattle. Some taxonomists, however, think it is merely a variant of *Actinomyces odontolyticus.*

Arachnia

This genus is represented by only one species *Arachnia propionica,* an organism that resembles *Actinomyces israelii* but is different in its cell wall composition and in the production of propionic acid from the fermentation of glucose. It is an oral commensal and opportunistic pathogen.

Eubacterium

Organisms of this genus colonise dental plaque and much of the digestive tract. *Eubacterium alactolyticum* and *saburreum* are the dominant oral species. They are non-sporing anaerobic rods.

Propionibacterium

Members of this genus could best be described as anaerobic diphtheroids. They are characterised by the production of propionic acid from the breakdown of carbohydrates. They are isolated predominantly from dental plaque.

Bacterionema

Bacterionema matruchotii is a short Gram-positive rod possessing a long curved filamentous appendage. It grows well in aerobic conditions as well as anaerobic and is found in dental plaque and calculus. Some authorities now regard this organism as a member of the genus *Corynebacterium* (Plate 5).

Rothia

Rothia dentocariosa is a pleomorphic Gram-positive filament that may appear coccal in older cultures. The organism has been isolated from carious dentine and dental plaque.

Bifidobacterium

Bifidobacteria are anaerobic Y-branching, Gram-positive rods resembling lactobacilli. They are very early colonisers of the digestive tract and are regular inhabitants of the oral cavity of infants. They may become established in dental plaque in adults.

Clostridium

Clostridia are spore-forming, Gram-positive anaerobic rods that are regarded as transient in the human mouth. Many clostridia inhabit the lower digestive tract of man. There are a few reports of the isolation of commensal clostridia from the mouths of patients in long-stay hospitals.

Gram-negative rods and filaments

Considerable interest has been generated into the association of Gram-negative bacteria with periodontal disease and this has produced corresponding modifications to the classification of these organisms. Improved sampling and cultural techniques have enabled a much more detailed study of the anaerobes resident in dental plaque and the gingival crevice. A list of genera of Gram-negative rods and filaments found in the mouth is given in Table 12.4.

Haemophilus

Members of the genus *Haemophilus* are indigenous to the upper respiratory tract of man. In saliva the predominant species are *Haemophilus influenzae* and *parainfluenzae* but in dental plaque *Haemophilus segnis* is most commonly isolated. *Haemophilus aphrophilus* may also be present. It is thought that these organisms are of low pathogenicity in the oral cavity.

TABLE 12.4. Gram-negative rods and filaments found in the mouth.

Genus	Atmosphere for growth
Haemophilus	Aerobic
Eikenella	Aerobic + CO_2
Campylobacter (Vibrio)	Microaerophilic + CO_2
Bacteroides	Anaerobic + CO_2
Fusobacterium	Anaerobic
Leptotrichia	Anaerobic
Actinobacillus	Microaerophilic + CO_2
Capnocytophaga	Aerobic + CO_2
Wolinella	Anaerobic
Selenomonas	Anaerobic
Coliforms (Escherichia) (Proteus) (Klebsiella)	Aerobic

Eikenella

This genus is represented by one species *Eikenella corrodens* which characteristically produces colonies that pit the surface of the agar. These organisms are Gram-negative rods resembling *Bacteroides* but are able to grow in air supplemented with carbon dioxide. They have been implicated in endocarditis and brain abscesses but their role as oral pathogens is not clear; they are commensals of the gingival crevice.

Campylobacter (Vibrio)

Comma-shaped motile Gram-negative bacilli that grow in air are mostly classified as *Vibrio* spp. Similar organisms that grow microaerophilically (5-6% O_2), usually with supplemented CO_2, are classified currently as *Campylobacter* spp. *Campylobacter sputorum* and *concisus* are found in dental plaque and the gingival crevice. Although relatively little is known about these organisms a significant increase in counts of *Campylobacter sputorum* with increasing gingival index has been reported.

Bacteroides

There are many species of the genus *Bacteroides* in the mouth. The taxonomy of the group is difficult and the role of these organisms in disease is not yet clear. *Bacteroides* are strictly anaerobic Gram-negative bacteria often exhibiting pleomorphism ranging from long filaments to almost coccal forms. Table 12.5 lists some of the currently accepted species and sub-species of oral bacteroides.

As with other strict anaerobes the favoured habitat of *Bacteroides* in the mouth is the gingival crevice and

TABLE 12.5 Oral bacteroides

Species	Black pigment
Saccharolytic	
Bacteroides melaninogenicus ss *melaninogenicus*	+
B. intermedius	+
B. denticola	+
B. loescheii	+
B. buccalis	−
B. pentosaceus	−
B. oralis	
B. buccale/capillus	−
B. oris	−
Asaccharolytic	
B. gingivalis	+
B. asaccharolyticus	+
B. levii	+
B. ureolyticus	−

dental plaque. In healthy mouths few, if any, asaccharolytic strains are isolated and *Bacteroides melaninogenicus* ss *intermedius* and ss *melaninogenicus* predominate. These organisms produce black-pigmented colonies when grown on blood-containing media, a distinguishing feature that has helped in the study of these organisms as part of the complex gingival flora (Plates 1 & 2). Similar, but non-pigmented, organisms can be isolated from the same sites and these have been given a variety of names reflecting the taxonomic confusion (for example, *Bacteroides oralis* and *ruminicola*). *Bacteroides loescheii*, *denticola* and *levii* have recently been given species status but little about them is yet known. Asaccharolytic bacteroides increase in periodontal disease (Chap. 14) where *Bacteroides gingivalis* is the most common isolate. *Bacteroides asaccharolyticus* is found in the vagina and digestive tract but is rare in the mouth. Little is yet known about *Bacteroides capillus* or *levii* in the mouth.

Medical microbiologists are mostly concerned with a group of saccharolytic, non-pigmented bacteroides that are considerably less fastidious than the oral strains. *Bacteroides fragilis*, *thetaiotaomicron* and related species are perhaps the most numerous bacteria of the large bowel but they are rarely reported from the mouth and probably only occur as transients.

Fusobacterium

Fusobacteria are Gram-negative, strictly anaerobic filamentous bacteria whose filaments generally have pointed ends (Plate 3). On blood agar the colonies have an indefinite, even rhizoid, edge. Initially two species were recognised in the mouth, *Fusobacterium nucleatum* and *polymorphum* but these have been found to be so similar that they have now been put together in one species – *nucleatum*. Fusobacteria are isolated from the gingival crevice and dental plaque.

Leptotrichia

Leptotrichia buccalis is the only species in this genus. The organism is an oral commensal previously classified with the fusobacteria but differing from them in many biochemical tests. *Leptotrichia buccalis* is a stout filament with at least one pointed end (Plate 4). The colonies resemble those of fusobacteria but are larger. It is frequently seen on smears taken from the gingival margin in acute necrotising ulcerative gingivitis (Chap. 15 and Plate 7) but is probably present in small numbers in the gingival crevice of healthy mouths.

Actinobacillus

The organism *Actinobacillus actinomycetemcomitans* is of very uncertain affiliation as it differs considerably from other members of the genus *Actinobacillus* that are important animal pathogens. In the mouth *Actinobacillus actinomycetemcomitans* is found as a commensal in small numbers in the gingival crevice (Plate 9).

Capnocytophaga

The genus *Capnocytophaga* contains three species *Capnocytophaga ochracea*, *sputigena* and *gingivalis*. All are isolated from dental plaque and the gingival crevice of healthy subjects. These organisms are Gram-negative rods that have fastidious growth requirements and will only grow in an atmosphere containing increased CO_2. Some of the strains studied produce colonies with a spreading edge; others pit the agar and are firmly adherent. This property is dependent on growth conditions and media. Many strains exhibit a so-called 'gliding motility' when wet-film preparations are viewed under dark-ground or phase-contrast microscopy. Some early papers reporting similar organisms often refer to them as 'gliding bacilli' or '*Fusobacterium girans*'. (Plate 8)

Wolinella

Wolinella succinogenes is the name recently ascribed to the Gram-negative, comma-shaped bacillus *Vibrio succinogenes*. This pathogen of the intestine of pigs is found as a commensal of the oral cavity of man. Some workers have found that most oral vibrios resemble *Wolinella (Vibrio) succinogenes*, whereas others find that their isolates resemble *Campylobacter (Vibrio) sputorum*. These organisms are found predominantly in the gingival crevice and their numbers have been reported to increase in periodontal disease. A second species *Wolinella recta* has been identified as a member of the flora of the gingival crevice.

Selenomonas

It is disputed whether the organism *Selenomonas sputigena* is a protozoon or a bacterium although current thinking favours the latter. It is a Gram-negative, curved rod with tufts of flagella arising from the inner aspect of the curve. The organism is found in dental plaque, calculus and in the gingival crevice.

Coliforms

Although much of the digestive tract supports a coliform flora few such Gram-negative aerobic bacilli are isolated from the mouth. Usually they are regarded as transients although *Proteus* spp, *Klebsiella* spp and *Escherichia coli* may remain in the mouth for some months. They are not known to cause any oral disease. Most will be transmitted to the mouth by a faecal-oral route either directly or on food. *Klebsiella* spp may become established in the mouths of debilitated patients and some denture wearers but this does not seem to produce any ill effects.

Spirochaetes

These strictly anaerobic organisms are isolated from the deeper parts of the gingival crevice and are the last organisms to appear in the developing oral flora. Spirochaetes are nutritionally demanding as well as being dependent for growth on the lowest oxidation-reduction potential of any of the oral bacteria. Two genera are present in the mouth, *Borrelia* and *Treponema*. Although some oral spirochaetes can now be cultured on very rich media most are detected only by dark-ground or phase-contrast microscopy. This has produced a confusing classification based on highly variable microscopic appearances. Oral spirochaetes are narrow, helically coiled with pointed ends. They are motile and stain Gram-negative but are difficult to see unless stained by a silver-impregnation method. The larger and less tightly coiled spirochaetes seen in oral specimens were termed *Borrelia vincenti* and *Borrelia buccale*. Current classification includes these organisms in the

genus *Treponema*, as *Treponema vincenti* and *buccale*. Other treponemes are smaller and more tightly coiled and include *macrodentium, orale* and *denticola*. Improved cultural and serological techniques may soon improve understanding of these demanding organisms.

Yeasts

About 30 per cent of the adult population carry yeasts as part of their normal oral flora. These are usually situated on the hard palate, dorsum of the tongue and in the upper buccal sulcus. Denture wearers may have an increased carriage rate of yeasts. The most common yeast isolated from the mouth is *Candida albicans* but *Candida tropicalis, krusei* and *parapsilosus* and *Torulopsis glabrata* have also been isolated; others may be carried as commensals in a small proportion of individuals (Fig 12.2).

Mycoplasma

Two mycoplasmas *Mycoplasma orale* and *salivarium* are found in the mouth, usually in the gingival crevice but also in dental plaque. Both grow readily in anaerobic conditions but poorly in air and *orale* is the more fastidious of the two. Two further species, *faucium* and *buccale*, are now thought to be variants of *Mycoplasma orale*. These organisms appear to be ubiquitous oral commensals and although sporadic reports link mycoplasmas to the progression of periodontal disease the evidence is far from convincing at present.

Protozoa

Two protozoons, *Entamoeba gingivalis* and *Trichomonas tenax*, are regularly isolated from the mouth, particularly from the gingival crevice. About 25 per cent of subjects in the U.S.A. carry these oral protozoa as commensals in disease-free mouths. In severe periodontal disease the isolation rate has been as high as 100 per cent in some studies but no pathogenic role has been ascribed to these protozoa in the mouth.

Viruses

Viruses are obligate parasites and it is perhaps incorrect to regard any of them as commensal but undoubtedly the 'normal' microbial flora of most adults will contain herpes simplex virus. The virus lies dormant in neural tissue and periodically migrates along sensory nerves to the perioral skin mucosa where the characteristic lesions of secondary herpes

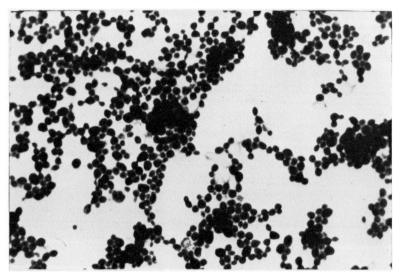

FIG. 12.2. Blastospores of *Candida albicans*.

may be seen. Non-disease-associated adenoviruses may be isolated from the throat and are perhaps best regarded as transients. Most other viruses isolated from the mouth in the absence of disease for example cytomegalovirus, mumps virus and rubella virus are associated with subclinical infection or a prolonged convalescent period. Rabies virus may be present in the saliva of bats in the carrier state.

FURTHER READING

Hardie J.M. & Bowden G.H. (1974) The normal flora of the mouth. *In* Skinner F.A. & Carr J.G. eds. *The normal Microbial Flora of Man.* London. Academic Press.

van der Hoeven J.S. (1980) Microbial interactions in the mouth. *In* Lehner T. & Cimasoni G. eds. *The Borderland Between Caries and Periodontal Disease II.* London. Academic Press.

Marsh P.D. (1980) *Oral Microbiology.* Walton on Thames. Nelson.

Nord C–E. (1980) Anaerobic microorganisms in gingival plaque. *In* Lehner T. & Cimasoni G. (see above).

Socransky S.S. & Manganiello S.D. (1971) The oral microbiota of man from birth to senility. *Journal of Periodontology,* **42,** 485–94.

CHAPTER 13

Dental Plaque

In the absence of oral hygiene a deposit builds up on the surface of the tooth. This is called dental plaque and consists of bacteria, their extracellular products and glycoproteins. The innermost layers of this matrix adhere to the acquired pellicle covering the tooth, whereas the outer layers are loosely applied to the more tenacious mass of dental plaque. This outer layer, or *materia alba*, which comprises bacteria, squamous cells and food debris, is easily removed with a water spray, whereas the bulk of the deposit is not. Dental plaque imparts a rather matt appearance to the otherwise glossy enamel surface of the tooth but it is best seen after the use of a disclosing dye such erythrocin that stains the plaque red.

Dental plaque accumulates in areas of stagnation such as the gingival margin, interproximal spaces and occlusal fissures. Long-standing dental plaque may calcify to form calculus, especially in areas adjacent to the duct openings of the major salivary glands, notably on the buccal aspects of the upper molar teeth and the lingual aspects of the lower incisor teeth (Fig. 13.1).

Formation of dental plaque

In order to understand the development of dental plaque it is helpful to begin with a clean tooth surface and follow the development of the plaque that builds up in the absence of oral hygiene. In normal circumstances plaque is a dynamic entity, being constantly abraded by brushing or diet and building up in areas of stagnation. The following account

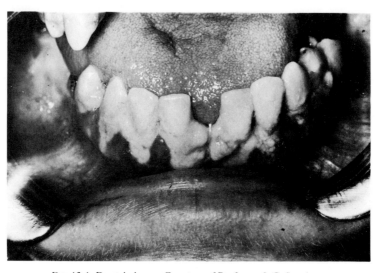

FIG. 13.1. Dental plaque. Courtesy of Professor J. C. Southam.

describes the formation of supragingival dental plaque; variations in this development occur in specialised areas such as the gingival crevice, occlusal fissure and interproximal space.

Pellicle

The acquired pellicle consists of glycoproteins derived from saliva. These are rapidly adsorbed on to any clean tooth surface in the mouth. According to a widely accepted theory the enzyme neuraminidase produced by a number of oral microorganisms, including *Bacteroides melaninogenicus* and *oralis*, and fusobacteria is involved. Neuraminidase splits sialic acid molecules off the glycoproteins, thereby altering the configuration of the glycoprotein molecule which then precipitates and adsorbs on to the enamel surface.

Early colonisation

Dental plaque builds up first in small defects or pits on the enamel surface and then spreads over the smooth surface. Bacteria become associated with the acquired glycoprotein pellicle almost immediately. The first organisms to attach include *Streptococcus sanguis*, other streptococci, and Gram-negative cocci (*Neisseria* and *Branhamella*). Most of these bacteria are derived from the salivary flora that bathes the tooth. After developing for about 24 hours, dental plaque consists largely of streptococci but a number of other genera are represented, notably *Neisseria*, *Branhamella*, *Veillonella*, *Corynebacterium*, *Actinomyces*, *Lactobacillus* and *Rothia*. Among the anaerobes *Veillonella* are the first to appear, followed by the facultative actinomycetes and the anaerobic *Actinomyces israelii*. As the plaque ages the numbers of anaerobes increase and after seven days fusobacteria and bacteroides can be detected. Initial oxidation-reduction potentials (Eh) of dental plaque may be +200 mV but by seven days the Eh has fallen to −110 mV or lower. The plaque becomes more filamentous and the numbers of streptococci, *Neisseria*, *Branhamella* and *Rothia* decline in relative terms.

Matrix

Dental plaque consists not only of bacteria but also of an organic matrix composed of precipitated salivary glycoprotein and extracellular polysaccharides derived from bacteria. These extracellular polysaccharides (glucans and levan) are produced by several species of oral streptococci, *Neisseria*, *Rothia* and some actinomycetes. Other material in the plaque matrix includes extracellular bacterial enzymes and diffusible waste products of bacterial metabolism.

Mature plaque

An important fact about mature dental plaque is the tremendous variation in its composition. A succession of microorganisms attaches to or becomes embedded in the plaque matrix. The development of the climax community of plaque is dependent on a number of microbial interactions; organisms produce factors that either enhance or inhibit the succession of other species in the plaque.

As the filaments in dental plaque increase they invade the deeper layers, giving the plaque the appearance of a pallisade when viewed in transmission electronmicrographs. This contrasts with the coccal appearance of early dental plaque (Figs. 13.2 and 13.3). The numbers of streptococci stabilise after around the 5th and 7th day and, as the overall num-

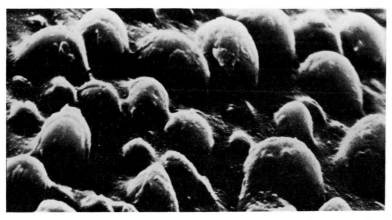

FIG. 13.2. Coccal appearance of early dental plaque. Scanning electronmicrograph, courtesy of Dr. C. A. Saxton.

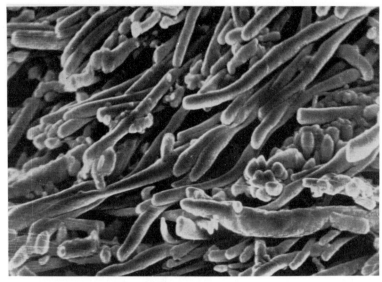

Fig. 13.3. Filaments invading deeper layers of dental plaque. Scanning electronmicrograph, courtesy of Dr. C. A. Saxton.

bers of organisms in the plaque increase, the relative proportion of the early coccal colonisers falls. The organisms usually found in mature, smooth surface dental plaque, between the 7th and 14th day, are shown in Table 13.1. Spirochaetes are found only in the most mature dental plaque because of their sensitivity to oxygen and fastidious nutritional requirements. They predominate at the apical border of the developing plaque, where the gingival margin protects the plaque from dislodging forces and a low Eh is thus established. As dental plaque ages, the deeper layers become deprived of oxygen and nutrients. Waste products of metabolism build up and there is a gradual reduction in the numbers of living organisms. Electronmicrographic studies show the presence of void spaces and disrupted bacteria.

TABLE 13.1. The principal organisms of mature dental plaque.

GRAM-POSITIVE COCCI
  Streptococcus sanguis
  Streptococcus mutans
  Streptococcus mitior
  Anaerobic streptococci

GRAM-NEGATIVE COCCI
  Neisseria
  Branhamella catarrhalis
  Veillonella parvula
  Veillonella alkalescens

GRAM-POSITIVE RODS AND FILAMENTS
  Actinomyces viscosus/naeslundii
  Actinomyces israelii
  Actinomyces odontolyticus
  Corynebacterium
  Bacterionema matruchotii
  Lactobacillus acidophilus
  Rothia dentocariosa
  Eubacterium

GRAM-NEGATIVE RODS AND FILAMENTS
  Bacteroides melaninogenicus
  Bacteroides intermedius
  Bacteroides oralis/ruminicola
  Bacteroides ureolyticus
  Leptotrichia buccalis
  Fusobacterium nucleatum
  Eikenella corrodens
  Haemophilus aphrophilus
  Haemophilus parainfluenzae
  Haemophilus segnis
  Capnocytophaga ochracea
  Campylobacter sputorum
  Wolinella succinogenes
  Wolinella recta
  Selenomonas sputigena

SPIROCHAETES
  Treponema macrodentium
  Treponema orale

PROTOZOA
  Entamoeba gingivalis
  Trichomonas tenax

Microbial interactions in dental plaque

With such a density of microorganisms it follows that there are many microbial interactions in dental plaque; these may be beneficial or detrimental to the constituent bacteria. Fig. 13.4 illustrates a close association of bacteria; streptococci are arranged along a filament of the organism *Bacterionema matruchotii* to form bodies known as 'corn-cobs'. The importance *in vivo* of many of the microbial interactions studied *in vitro* is difficult to determine.

species such as *Bacteroides*, *Actinomyces israelii* and anaerobic cocci. Also, the extracellular polysaccharides produced by streptococci, *Neisseria* and actinomycetes can be utilised as an energy source for related species and unrelated species such as *Lactobacillus*. Such polysaccharides also form part of the sticky matrix which enables some bacteria to resist detachment from the plaque.

There are growth factors such as vitamin K produced by corynebacteria that stimulate the growth

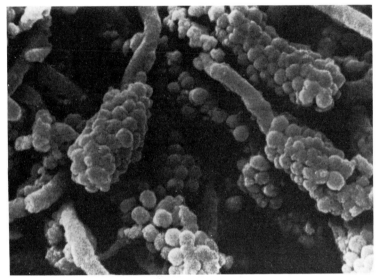

FIG. 13.4. 'Corn cobs'. Scanning electronmicrograph, courtesy of Dr. C. A. Saxton.

Bacteria that lower the pH by the fermentation of carbohydrates including *Streptococcus mutans*, *sanguis* and lactobacilli, produce an environment unsuitable for the multiplication of organisms that are intolerant of a very low pH, such as *Veillonella* or *Bacteroides*.

Bacterial metabolism may produce substances harmful to other bacteria. Hydrogen peroxide, for example, produced by *Streptococcus mutans* and *mitior* inhibits actinomycetes and a wide range of other oral organisms. In addition, inhibitory substances termed bacteriocins which are produced by most oral streptococci and bacteroides inhibit other strains of the same or related species *in vitro*, and may play a role as an ecological determinant *in vivo*.

On the other hand, some microbial interactions are beneficial to various organisms. For example, bacterial metabolism may reduce the Eh in the micro-environment enabling the multiplication of anaerobic

of *Bacteroides melaninogenicus*. Some bacteria, notably bacteroides, can utilise succinate by-products of bacterial metabolism and *Streptococcus sanguis* supports the growth of *Streptococcus mutans* by the production of para-amino-benzoic acid. Spiro chaetes, as well as requiring a low Eh, are also stimulated by the production of fatty acids by fusobacteria and bacteroides. One interesting utilisation of a bacterial metabolic product is that shown by *Veillonella* which can metabolise the lactate produced by streptococci and thus reduce the fall in pH that would be inhibitory to them.

Variations in dental plaque

The dynamic nature of dental plaque is one of its most interesting features but this also makes impossible any definitive statement about its composition. Marked variation may occur at any one site on a particular tooth sampled on different occasions, and indeed sites on the same tooth only 1 mm apart have been shown to differ in microbial composition in a striking way. The quantity and nature of dental plaque at different sites on one tooth and on different teeth in the mouth may vary even more widely, as may variations in plaque composition in different subjects. Although dental plaque may build up extraordinarily in relation to restorations or misplaced teeth, a consideration of normal teeth in a normal arch provides markedly different anatomical sites each of which is associated with characteristic plaques. These sites include: supragingival smooth surfaces (buccal, palatal and lingual); subgingival; approximal; and occlusal pit and fissure.

(1) Smooth surface plaque (supragingival): (see above)

(2) Subgingival plaque. The protection of the gingival tissues ensures that deposits of plaque are much less affected by changes in the oral environment. The matrix has more epithelial squames and pus cells than are found supragingivally and immunoglobulins are also present. Because the fall in Eh is achieved more rapidly in this protected environment, the plaque 'matures' faster than supragingival plaque so that a three-day old subgingival plaque may resemble that of a 14-day old supragingival plaque. The most important microbial distinction between the two plaques is the presence and numbers of anaerobes. Spirochaetes, anaerobic cocci and asaccharolytic bacteroides are usually found only in the subgingival plaque.

(3) Approximal plaque. Some detailed and elegant studies have shown considerable variations in the composition of approximal plaque. *Actinomyces viscosus/naeslundii* is the predominant organism, followed by *Actinomyces israelii*. *Streptococcus sanguis* is the most common streptococcus but some studies have shown that certain subjects may harbour large numbers of *Streptococcus mutans*. Lactobacilli are usually isolated, although they can be consistently absent from some subjects. *Veillonella* and various Gram-negative anaerobic rods complete the list of dominant organisms.

(4) Occlusal pit and fissure plaque. Although artificial fissures have been inserted in mouths to facilitate the study of occlusal fissure plaque, few studies of natural fissures have been reported. The deepest parts of occlusal fissures contain few viable bacteria and numerous dead cells. More occlusally, the plaque consists of coccal cells with fewer filaments than are seen in smooth surface plaque. *Streptococcus*

sanguis and *mutans* are found in addition to *salivarius* which is not a feature of other plaques. Corynebacteria and *Veillonella* are present in higher proportions than in other plaques. Electron-microscope studies have shown that some of the densely packed bacteria in occlusal fissure plaque contain intracellular polysaccharide granules but there is little extracellular matrix.

Calculus

Calculus is produced by the calcification of supra and subgingival dental plaque. As the calcium phosphate deposits are often patchy hardness varies. Dental plaque may cover the established layer of calculus and calcify, building up a thicker layer of calculus. Saliva contains a super-saturated solution of calcium and phosphate and several mechanisms for calcification have been proposed, including local pH changes and 'seeding' on crystals or small particles. The Gram-positive rod *Bacterionema matruchotii* (Plate 5) may play an important role in promoting the calcification of dental plaque, as well as a number of Gram-negative organisms such as *Veillonella, Neisseria, Haemophilus* and *Bacteroides*.

Calculus contains a large variety of organisms, 22 species of bacteria having been cultivated from disrupted samples of calculus. *Streptococcus sanguis, mitior* and actinomycetes predominate, and fuso-bacteria, *Bacteroides melaninogenicus, Leptotrichia buccalis* and *Neisseria* are also very common. *Selenomonas* spp have also been isolated in relatively large numbers from many calculus samples.

Investigation of dental plaque

Attempts to study dental plaque have met with many difficulties. Quantitative studies require accurate weighing of very small samples and the error in this can be considerable. The time taken to weigh a sample often leads to death of some organisms and consequent distortion of the results of viable count studies. As described previously, many anaerobic organisms are found in plaque and several pre-cautions have been introduced to prevent aeration of the specimen which would then reduce the viability of anaerobes and alter the relative proportion of viable organisms in the specimen. Precautions can be taken which involve sampling tools connected to a supply of oxygen-free gas that flows over the plaque *in situ* and over the sample as it is transferred to transport or culture media.

In addition, removal of a sample from the mouth will often alter the stimuli and constraints to bacterial growth, affecting the proportion of organisms in the final cultures. Transporting organisms to the laboratory is another area where error can occur and none of the transport media so far developed can replace the value of immediate culture. Some plaque samples may be partially calcified and will require some form of dispersion before culturing. Mechanical, enzymatic and ultrasonic dispersion methods have all been adopted but all reduce the viability of certain organisms; failure to disperse a sample in a small volume of fluid will reduce the total viable count. Gram-negative filaments are particularly sensitive to ultrasonic disruption and all anaerobes are sensitive to the essential delays involved in disrupting the sample.

Culture systems for anaerobes vary considerably. These include anaerobic cabinets, anaerobic jars and anaerobic roll-tubes (the Hungate system). Each has its advantages and drawbacks. Specimens may be cultured on selective or non-selective media and may be diluted to a greater or lesser degree. Selective media may reduce the yield of a given organism but may facilitate the isolation of species present in small numbers that would otherwise be missed. Excessive dilution of the sample may result in an organism, though present, failing to grow.

Even with successful isolation and quantitation the identity of some organisms found in dental plaque remains in doubt or in dispute. New organisms are being identified but there is still confusion about the taxonomic position of some of these. There has been considerable progress, however, in the understanding of the developments and structure of dental plaque, although much still remains to be elucidated.

Effects of dental plaque

Dental plaque is involved in the aetiology of dental caries and periodontal disease, and *Streptococcus sanguis* and *mutans* found in dental plaque have been implicated in many cases of infective endocarditis (see Chaps. 14 and 17).

Control of dental plaque

Diet. Much of the current development of preventive dentistry is aimed at the control of dental plaque because it is reasoned that control of plaque will control caries and periodontal disease. The first prerequisite is dietary control. Plaque increases considerably in the presence of carbohydrate, especially sucrose. Limiting dietary carbohydrate has a dramatic effect on plaque volume.

Physical removal. Oral hygiene instruction is directed at physical removal of plaque by tooth brushing, the use of dental floss, inter-dental wooden wedges and other devices. Disclosing the presence of dental plaque with dyes such as erythrocin helps pick out the areas where plaque has built up.

Ultrasonic scaling devices. These remove plaque mechanically and also provide a brisk flushing action from the water spray. As well as dislodging plaque and calculus the ultrasonic vibration may disrupt bacteria in the subgingival plaque.

Antiseptics. Considerable attention has been paid to chlorhexidine, but less so to povidone-iodine. Both antiseptics reduce the number of plaque bacteria. Chlorhexidine binds to the glycoprotein pellicle and thus adsorbed it is able to act for a number of hours. Gram-positive organisms are most sensitive. Plaque is effectively reduced and any that does accumulate usually appears immature, with a few coccal colonies on the glycoprotein pellicle. Few organisms develop resistance and superinfection is rare even in patients who have received chlorhexidine for long periods.

Antibiotics. After initial failures in the 1960's the use of antibiotics as agents for controlling plaque was largely discontinued, although recent proposals that a variety of specific organisms may play a major role in both chronic adult periodontal disease and juvenile periodontal disease has led to an upsurge of interest in using antibiotics to control dental plaque. So far the results are not encouraging. Antibiotic therapy rarely succeeds in reducing numbers of organisms for long periods. Resistant strains may develop or there may be superinfection with other resistant bacteria and for these reasons antibiotics cannot be recommended.

FURTHER READING

Bowden G.H. & Hardie J.M. (1975) Microbial variations in approximal dental plaque. *Caries Research,* **9,** 253–77.

Leach S.A. (1977) Mode of action of chlorhexidine in the mouth. *In* Lehner T. ed. *The Borderland between Caries and Periodontal Disease.* London, Academic Press.

Marsh P. (1980) *Oral Microbiology.* Walton-on-Thames, Nelson.

McHugh, W.D. (1970) *Dental Plaque.* Edinburgh, E. & S. Livingstone.

Newman H.N. (1977) Ultrastructure of the apical border of dental plaque. *In* Lehner T. ed. *The Borderland between Caries and Periodontal Disease.* London, Academic Press.

Newman H.N. & Poole D.F. (1974) Structural and ecological aspects of dental plaque. *In* Skinner F.A. & Carr J.G. eds, *The Normal Microbial Flora of Man.* Society for Applied Microbiology, Symposium 3. London, Academic Press.

Sidaway D.A. (1978) A microbiological study of dental calculus. *Journal of Periodontal Research,* **13,** 349-66.

Williams R.A.D. & Elliot J.C. (1979) *Basic and Applied Dental Biochemistry.* Edinburgh, Churchill Livingstone.

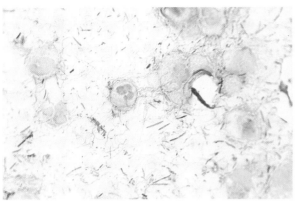

PLATE 7. Gram stain of gingival debris from Vincent's gingivitis showing pus cells, spirochaetes, large Gram-negative rods and smaller pleomorphic Gram-negative bacteria.

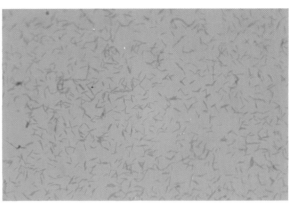

PLATE 8. Gram stain of *Capnocytophaga ochracea* showing pale-staining, Gram-negative rods.

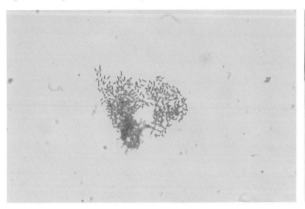

PLATE 9. Gram stain of *Actinobacillus actinomycetemcomitans* showing Gram-negative coccobacilli.

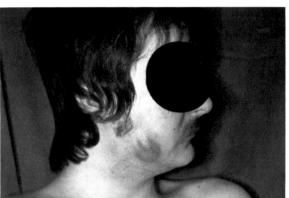

PLATE 10. Clinical appearance of actinomycosis.

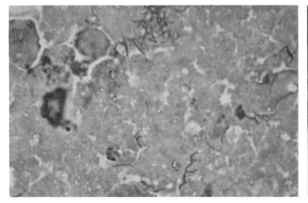

PLATE 11. Gram stain of pus from actinomycosis to show Gram-positive branching filaments.

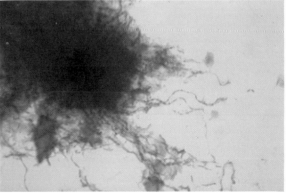

PLATE 12. Gram stain of a compressed sulphur granule showing the mass of branching filaments of *Actinomyces israelii* that compose the sulphur granule.

CHAPTER 14

Dental Caries and Periodontal Disease

These two major disease processes of the oral tissues have more in common than was previously thought. Dental plaque harbours microorganisms that have been implicated directly or indirectly in the aetiology of both conditions and furthermore methods of preventing both dental diseases have largely concentrated on controlling dental plaque. It is likely that future research will illustrate further the inter-relationship between these two conditions.

DENTAL CARIES (Fig. 14.1)

History

Many theories of dental caries have been postulated. It has been suggested that the irreversible destruction of the hard dental tissues was the result of chelation of the calcium salts, proteolysis of the enamel sheaths and dissociation of the enamel. In 1890 Miller postulated his chemico-parasitic theory of tooth decay which drew on his earlier work and the work of others who had noted the accumulation of bacteria on the teeth. Miller's theory suggested that these bacteria fermented dietary carbohydrate to produce lactic acid among other acids which then destroyed the tooth substance. This latter theory is the one which has stood the test of subsequent experiments.

Bacteria that could produce acids, particularly lactic acid, and could tolerate conditions of low pH ($\leq$ 5.0) were those mostly suspected of initiating caries. Although in 1924 Clarke discovered *Streptococcus mutans* in deep carious lesions, most attention was paid to members of the genus *Lactobacillus*. In 1954-55 Orland and his co-workers reported experi-

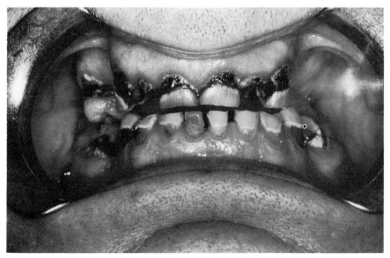

FIG. 14.1. Grossly carious teeth. Courtesy of Professor J. C. Southam.

ments in which germ-free (gnotobiotic) rats were fed a diet rich in carbohydrate; these test animals were monoinfected with enterococci and developed caries. Control animals were kept germ-free and did not develop caries. Subsequent experiments of a similar nature were performed in many centres and with a variety of rodents and it became clear that *Streptococcus mutans* was the most cariogenic organism known and that in monoinfections lactobacilli possessed little cariogenic activity.

Streptococcus mutans and dental caries

Since the early experiments a vast literature on the association of *Streptococcus mutans* with dental caries has appeared. Sucrose seems to enhance the cariogenicity, probably by providing substrate for acid production and by increasing the amount of sticky plaque which will allow larger numbers of bacteria to attach to the tooth. Further experiments have extended the study of *Streptococcus mutans* in caries initiation in hamsters, gerbils and later monkeys and other primates. It is now clear that strains found to be particularly cariogenic in one species are not necessarily so in another. Furthermore the complex nature of the microbial flora of dental plaque is far removed from the simple experiments involving only a single strain in an otherwise germ-free mouth. Few experiments involving mixed cultures have yet been undertaken and because of the complexity of *in vivo* work further advances are likely to come from *in vitro* cultures in artificial mouths or chemostats.

Streptococcus mutans is divided into several serotypes (a–g); c and d are the prevalent serotypes in Europe and the U.S.A. These serotypes may be of different cariogenicity for man but firm evidence for this is not yet available.

Other cariogenic organisms

Much of the work on the association of other organisms with caries has centred on studies on germ-free animals. In this way some strains of *Streptococcus sanguis, mitior, milleri* and *salivarius* have been shown to have cariogenic potential in certain animal model systems. *Lactobacillus casei* and *acidophilus* have caused caries in gnotobiotic rats. *Actinomyces viscosus/naeslundii* causes root surface caries in rats as well as periodontal disease.

Caries in man

It is tempting to extrapolate to man the findings of experiments with gnotobiotic animals. Human studies are far more complex because of the presence of normal mixed microbial flora. Many extensive studies have shown an increased number of *Streptococcus mutans* in subjects with active caries. This may reflect a true pathogenic role for the organism or demonstrate that the organism multiplies rapidly in the lesion once it has been initiated. Laborious and technically demanding longitudinal studies have attempted to show changes with time in the microbial flora of a particular tooth surface, as it progresses from normality to decay. Just after a surface becomes carious, as detected radiographically, there is an increase in the numbers of *Streptococcus mutans*. This would suggest that other microorganisms, alone or in combination, initiate the lesion and that the acid produced by *Streptococcus mutans* establishes the lesion and extends it.

A major difficulty encountered in any human caries study is that of early detection of the lesion. By the time a lesion is visible radiographically it is already large enough for several microbial successions to have occurred after the initiation of the lesion. If tooth enamel is partially decalcified and then recalcified constantly, as some workers suggest, then caries would be initiated when the decalcification was too great for any subsequent total recalcification. Microbial changes may then occur in this altered and more retentive site that lead to the production of an established carious lesion.

In human studies the association of *Streptococcus sanguis* and *mitior* with human caries has been postulated on the basis of their acid production and acid tolerance, their presence in dental plaque, in addition to the somewhat arbitrary extrapolation from animal studies. Lactobacilli are only present in dental plaque in small numbers and their aetiological role in caries initiation is doubted for this reason. Lactobacilli may, however, play a considerable role in the acid-destruction of dentine in the established lesion. *Actinomyces viscosus/naeslundii* has been isolated in large numbers from root surface carious lesions in man and from gingival plaque at the neck of the tooth. It is known to initiate caries of the root surface in rats and may well do so in humans. The existence of large numbers of *Actinomyces* in approximal plaque, often dominating *Streptococcus mutans*, has increased the index of suspicion that these are cariogenic organisms in man.

The established carious lesion

From the earliest studies of Miller many types of bacteria have been demonstrated in the dentinal tubules of the advancing carious lesion (Plate 6).

Protected from forces of detachment it is easy to appreciate that even non-adherent organisms may contribute to the destruction of dentine. Proteolytic action may also play a part in this tissue which is less calcified than enamel. Studies have usually been carried out on extracted teeth sampled from the pulp chamber to the outer areas of the lesion, thus avoiding contamination with oral organisms. The flora of the advancing lesion is often complex and invariably contains more than one genus. Even the early photomicrographs of Miller showed this in 1890. Lactobacilli and streptococci are the predominant organisms in most studies, but Gram-positive rods and filaments for example *Bifidobacterium, Propionibacterium, Eubacterium, Actinomyces* and *Arachnia* are also reported from the few studies that used good anaerobic techniques.

Infection of the pulp

As the carious lesion progresses the pulp becomes inflamed, either as a result of the direct invasion of bacteria or the effect of their diffusible products. The inflammatory response, termed pulpitis, may result in the pulp becoming necrotic. Increasing pressure from the build-up of pus in the pulp forces organisms out of the apex of the root where a periapical lesion becomes established. This periapical osteitis may extend until the periostium of the alveolus is involved, producing the swelling of a dental abscess. If left unchecked the abscess will discharge pus into the mouth or through the facial skin. Rarely pus will track along the fascial planes.

Almost all early studies of dental abscesses and pulpal infections involved samples of pus collected whilst draining over the skin or mucosae. Recent studies using aspirates of pus and good anaerobic techniques have given a completely different impression of the flora of the dental abscess. Early studies reported the *'Streptococcus viridans'* group of organisms as being the most common. A few other aerobic species were mentioned and *Veillonella* was the only anaerobe commonly reported. Recently it has been shown that most dental abscesses contain a mixture of organisms with anaerobes predominating, such as anaerobic cocci, *Actinomyces, Bacteroides melaninogenicus* and *gingivalis* and *Veillonella* spp.

Bacteriological sampling

Sampling from carious lesions is of no diagnostic value.

Infected root canals are often sampled with paper points as part of endodontic therapy. Quantitation of the bacteria present is probably of more value than speciation but the samples taken usually make this impossible. Paper points are inserted carefully into the root canal, removed and placed in a transport fluid or culture broth. After incubation the broth is subcultured and organisms indentified. If the point is not placed in a transport medium the specimen will rapidly dry out. Samples directly plated at the chairside may be most useful and give semi-quantitative results. It may be helpful to know the nature of infecting organisms in problem cases but in general a good endodontic technique with disinfectant irrigation should be adequate and bacteriology will add little. However, sampling of root canals during therapy has an educational value for students who can check their aseptic technique and, if semi-quantitation is available, can check that the bacterial counts indeed fall. Many teaching units retain endodontic sampling for this reason.

Dental abscesses should be sampled by aspiration and the syringe, with needle suitably protected, sent to the laboratory. Special anaerobic transport systems using gassed tubes may be available (Chap. 10).

Microbiological aspects of caries prevention

Diet

Restriction of dietary sucrose reduces the substrate available to plaque bacteria. The amount of acid produced in plaque is less if sucrose substitutes are used and there is some evidence that caries rates fall as a result of the reduction in sucrose intake. The form in which sucrose is taken is also important as sticky retentive sweet foods remain in the mouth much longer and are more completely metabolised by oral bacteria than sucrose drinks which are rapidly swallowed.

Plaque control

Fluoride. Although fluoride is largely regarded as reducing the solubility of enamel and thus increasing resistance to acid attack, it is also an antibacterial agent. Evidence is so far unclear but it may be that fluoride levels in plaque achieve concentrations that inhibit acid-producing bacteria. This effect may be brought about by altering the total mass of plaque or by changing its composition.

Chlorhexidine and povidone-iodine have been used as anti-plaque agents but studies on their uses have concentrated largely on reduction of periodontal disease. There is some evidence, however, that daily rinsing with chlorhexidinc will reduce the incidence of caries on smooth surfaces.

Enzymes. Dextranase and mutanase break down plaque matrix but have not been found particularly effective.

Toothbrushing. This and other physical means of plaque removal can control the development of smooth surface caries by reducing the mass of bacterial plaque that accumulates. It is much more difficult to remove plaque adequately from occlusal fissures and approximal surfaces to prevent caries.

Antibiotics. Use of antibiotics in humans will lead to the emergence of resistant strains and antibiotics with important uses elsewhere in the body will become useless as resistance develops. Antibiotics must be condemned as anti-plaque agents.

Immunisation against dental caries

Prevention of dental caries by immunisation is based on the belief that most carious lesions in man are initiated by *Streptococcus mutans.* Work has centred on the production of a vaccine to *Streptococcus mutans* that will stimulate the production of antibodies to the organism which can then reach the sites where caries is likely to develop and so exert a protective effect.

Antibodies in caries. Secretory IgA (sIgA) to *Streptococcus mutans* appears to rise in the saliva of those with increased caries experience, whereas caries-free subjects appear to have only low levels of specific sIgA. Serum IgG and IgM to *Streptococcus mutans* rise in active caries but if the lesion is filled or the tooth extracted IgG and IgM levels decline and sIgA levels in saliva increase. Although some of the antibody changes associated with caries are disputed it is clear that serum and salivary antibodies to *Streptococcus mutans* change with active caries experience. As tooth surfaces are avascular and the mouth is somewhat remote from systemic responses this is a very interesting and previously unsuspected phenomenon. The antibody response to *Streptococcus mutans* elicited by the host in normal circumstances is clearly not adequate to protect the human from the development of caries and studies on immunisation have sought to produce a means of stimulating the natural response into a protective one.

IgG antibodies and complement component C3 in saliva can opsonise *Streptococcus mutans* and cause the organism to be phagocytosed by the polymor-phonuclear leucocytes (PMNLs) that pass into saliva from the gingival crevice. By the time they reach the saliva, however, the viability and activity of PMNLs is much reduced. T-cell-mediated (Th and Ts) responses may also play a part in regulating the production of antibody by B-lymphocytes.

The vaccine. Various preparations of *Streptococcus mutans,* usually serotype c, have been used, including whole killed cells, living organisms and antigens derived from the cell wall of the bacterium. Vaccines have been developed from two cell-wall antigens, called proteins I and II or A and B. Further antigens have been derived from cell-wall enzymes such as glycosyltransferase. These vaccines have, so far, only been tried out in experimental animal studies, initially in rodents and later in monkeys. The protein antigens (I/II or A/B) have so far proved to be the most effective vaccines in protecting monkeys fed a cariogenic diet from developing caries. In some early studies the animals were infected with the strain from which the vaccine was derived but not so in later studies. Limited trials are under way in human volunteers using an oral vaccine containing whole killed cells.

Routes of administration. Parenteral administration, especially subcutaneous, has proved most effective. Submucosal and intravenous routes have also been used and the vaccine has been given orally. The protective effect of the vaccine has been related to an increase in the levels of IgG in serum and saliva rather than to a rise in local sIgA.

Caries reduction. Quite a major reduction in caries has been reported with some vaccines. In U.K. studies 60–80 per cent less caries was seen in immunised compared with sham-immunised monkeys. Counts of *Streptococcus mutans* in plaque also fell in the immunised monkeys.

Problems associated with immunisation against dental caries. Studies so far conducted into immunisation against dental caries have involved animals. It is thought that organisms other than *Streptococcus mutans* may play at least some part in human caries and the vaccine would not help prevent caries caused by these microorganisms. It is not clear how protective a vaccine derived from *Streptococcus mutans* serotype c would be against caries caused by other serotypes of the organism.

The vaccines at present in use are not sufficiently pure for parenteral use in humans. Some cross-reactivity between heart muscle and antibody to some protein components of the vaccine has been reported. This reaction is analogous to that seen in rheumatic fever following infection with Lancefield's group A beta-haemolytic streptococci, although in man *Streptococcus mutans* does not cause rheumatic fever. It does, however, indicate the need for further work in refining the vaccine.

Many vaccines carry a small risk of unwanted side-effects. In general however, the risk of contracting the usually serious disease or harmful sequelae is substantially higher than the likelihood of developing side effects to the vaccine, but if a dental caries vaccine is to be used successfully in humans it must be totally safe.

PERIODONTAL DISEASE

Periodontal disease can be classified as shown in Table 14.1.

TABLE 14.1. Classification of periodontal disease

ACUTE
    necrotising ulcerative gingivitis
    periodontal abscess
CHRONIC
    gingivitis
    periodontitis
    juvenile periodontitis (periodontosis)

Acute necrotising ulcerative gingivitis (Vincent's gingivitis)

The clinical appearance of this condition (Fig. 14.2) is characterised by the destruction of interdental papillae and often the gingival margin. It usually develops in patients with poor oral hygiene; additional stress for reasons not yet understood precipitates the development of the lesion. It is not uncommon in certain populations such as students and army recruits and it gained prominence in World War I when it was given the name of 'trench mouth'. Although early studies suggested that this was a transmissible bacterial infection no firm evidence for this has been put forward. There is however considerable evidence for this condition having an infective aetiology. Smears from the gingival crevice in the area show a characteristic appearance of pus cells. spiral organisms and large Gram-negative rods (Plate 7). Until the development of good anaerobic techniques these organisms could not be grown. Morphology alone was used to classify them as *Borrelia vincenti* and *Fusobacterium fusiforme* respectively. Ultrastructural and cultural studies later placed the spirochete with the genus *Treponema* as *Treponema vincenti*. *Fusobacterium fusiforme* has had a chequered career taxonomically and it now appears that the large cigar-shaped Gram-negative bacilli are *Leptotrichia buccalis*. Later cultural studies reported significant increases in *Bacteroides melaninogenicus*, *Vibrio* and *Campylobacter* spp in this form of gingivitis. *Treponema* spp, *Bacteroides melaninogenicus*

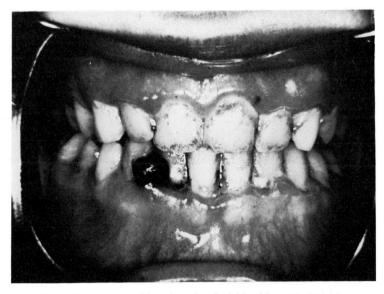

FIG. 14.2. Acute necrotising ulcerative gingivitis. (Vincent's gingivitis).

Treponema spp, *Bacteroides intermedius,* 'fusiforms' *Selenomonas* spp and a variety of other anaerobic and facultative organisms have been isolated from some subjects.

Few experimental animal studies have been undertaken with the flora from the lesions of acute necrotising ulcerative gingivitis. The potential for producing necrotising and ulcerative lesions on skin appears to reside with *Bacteroides melaninogenicus* and not with the spirochete or fusiform. Improved techniques for culturing spirochaetes are now available and this condition merits further study in the light of these technical advances.

Treatment

Metronidazole is the usual treatment for this condition although some clinicians especially in the U.S.A. prefer penicillin. Careful oral hygiene measures are also important.

Periodontal abscess

Few studies of the microflora of periodontal abscesses have been conducted. To avoid contamination of samples a shielded sampling tool should be used, and reduced transport media with good anaerobic methodology are essential for meaningful results. Gram-negative anaerobic rods predominate, especially *Bacteroides gingivalis,* but a wide range of species has been reported. Anaerobic cocci, facultative streptococci and *Actinomyces* are also found in large numbers in samples taken from the most apical region of the abscess. Perhaps significantly *Bacteroides gingivalis* is not a frequent isolate of the healthy gingival sulcus or of the early established pocket. The proteolytic activity of this organism may well contribute to its pathogenic potential.

Gingivitis

Inflammation of the gingivae appears to be caused by bacteria and their products in dental plaque adjacent to the gingival margin. There is an acute inflammatory response with dilatation of gingival capillaries and exudation of fluid containing immunoglobulins (IgG) complement and polymorphonuclear leucocytes. Removal of dental plaque leads to a resolution of gingivitis. No particular organisms have been implicated in gingivitis; it is more of a reaction to the mass of organisms and the products. Actinomycetes increase in numbers as do facultative and anaerobic cocci. Some animal studies have shown that mono-infection with *Actinomyces viscosus/naeslundii* can cause gingivitis.

Chronic periodontitis

The accumulation of bacteria and their products in the gingival sulcus leads initially to gingivitis and then, if not controlled, to periodontitis. In periodontitis the point of attachment of junctional epithelium to the tooth migrates apically and a gingival pocket forms. This deepened pocket is colonised by dental plaque bacteria and so a progressive deepening of the pocket ensues. In the advanced lesion the chronic inflammatory response leads to destruction of collagen and bone supporting the tooth. As it is a slow, progressive disease the severity of chronic periodontitis increases with age.

Not all the pathogenic mechanisms involved in periodontitis are understood. It seems likely that direct effects of microorganisms in dental plaque and host responses to some of these organisms, their products and to the components of plaque matrix, may all play some part in the destruction of the periodontium (Table 14.2).

TABLE 14.2. Microbial factors involved in periodontitis.

BACTERIA
    activation of classical complement pathway (Gram-positive)
    activation of alternative complement pathway (Gram-negative)

BACTERIAL ENZYMES
    collagenase
    hyaluronidase   } destruction of cells and increase in
    chondroitin sulphatase } permeability to bacterial products

BACTERIAL PRODUCTS AND PLAQUE COMPONENTS
    dextran
    levan   stimulation of lymphocytes (mostly
    endotoxin (Gram-   } B cells) leading to production of
            negative   antibody and lymphokines
            organisms)
    chemotactic factors: (Gram-positive organisms) — attraction of
                      polymorphonuclear leucocytes

Except for the behaviour of spirochaetes there is little evidence of bacterial invasion of the tissues from the base of the gingival pocket. It seems likely that enzymes produced by a variety of gingival bacteria increase the permeability of the epithelial lining to other components of plaque that in turn elicit inflammatory responses in the host (Table 14.3). Although a number of host responses to dental plaque could lead to destruction of the periodontal tissues it is by no means clear which mechanisms are involved. The chronic nature of the lesion suggests that a cell-mediated response may play an important part in the pathogenesis of the disease; immune complex, autoimmune and reaginic (IgE mediated) reactions have all been postulated. Perhaps the best evidence for the involvement of host responses in periodontitis is the reduced severity of the disease in patients with impaired immunity. An exception to this is the increased severity of gingivitis in patients with impaired polymorph function. Gingivitis is more severe in patients who take the drug levamisole that stimulates the immune responses.

TABLE 14.3. Host factors involved in periodontitis.

NON-SPECIFIC RESPONSES

(1) *Soluble mediators of inflammation*
  Complement activation (Gram-positive organisms in plaque)
  (endotoxin in Gram-negative organisms)
  Release of kinins, histamine and prostaglandins
  Attraction of polymorphonuclear leucocytes;
  (chemotactic factors from Gram-positive bacteria.)
(2) *Phagocytes*
  Polymorphonuclear phagocytes
  Macrophages
  Opsonisation by complement
(3) *Polyclonal B cell stimulation*
  By dextran, levan and endotoxins
(4) *Physical factors*
  Integrity of epithelium
  Flushing effect on gingival crevice fluid

SPECIFIC RESPONSES

  Antibody production (mostly IgG)
  Opsonisation by specific antibody
  Production of lymphokines from T-lymphocytes

Role of specific organisms

Considerable effort has gone into the search for specific organisms responsible for periodontitis. Quantitative studies of gingival pocket material have shown increased numbers, per gram of plaque, of a number of anaerobes especially *Bacteroides* spp. Advanced lesions harbour *Bacteroides gingivalis*, *Bacteroides ureolyticus (corrodens)*, *Eikenella corrodens* and spirochaetes in proportions far greater than in healthy gingival sulci. Most of these organisms are strict anaerobes and are very fastidious. It is therefore not surprising that their numbers increase only when the very reduced conditions in the depth of a pocket are established. Increased amounts of specific antibody to some bacteria have been reported, for example, *Bacteroides gingivalis*, *Bacteroides melaninogenicus* ss. *melaninogenicus*, *Actinomyces naeslundii* and *Treponema macrodentium*. Unfortunately high antibody levels can be found in control patients and so far their is no convincing evidence to link increased antibody production to an organism with the aetiology of the disease.

Lymphocyte transformation has been demonstrated to a number of diverse plaque bacteria including *Bacteroides melaninogenicus*, *Actinomyces viscosus/naeslundii*, *Actinomyces israelii* and *Veillonella alkalescens*. This diversity detracts from the concept of the possibility of one organism or type of organism being particularly peridontopathic.

An animal model of periodontitis using neutropaenic beagle dogs has shown that the junctional epithelium is first invaded by Gram-positive cocci and that Gram-positive organisms form the deepest bacterial layer of subgingival plaque. Gram-negative organisms, numerically dominant in subgingival plaque, are situated more coronally and may be attached to Gram-positive cocci and filaments that are in turn atached to the tooth. The inflammatory changes observed in gingivitis and periodontitis occur secondarily to this invasion by Gram-positive cocci. The shallow gingival pockets in dogs are not however directly comparable with the deep pockets in man which allow a more anaerobic flora to develop.

Treatment of periodontitis

The treatment of periodontitis depends largely on the control of dental plaque and the elimination of pockets that cannot be kept clean. Detailed descriptions of treatment are given in standard periodontology texts. Antibiotics have no place in this treatment, for reasons already mentioned. In severe lesions, however, instillation of antiseptics such as chlorhexidine may be helpful.

Juvenile periodontitis (periodontosis)

Some young patients develop a degree of periodontal destruction well in advance of that expected for their age. Although most immunological parameters appear normal there is evidence that production of macrophage migration inhibition factor is deficient. The search for a specific organism or organisms in this disease has shown that two organisms predominate in the gingival crevice flora of affected individuals; *Capnocytophaga ochracea* and *Actinobacillus actinomycetemcomitans* (Plates 8 & 9). These are periodontopathic in experimental animals and are usually found in only small numbers in gingival pockets of adults with periodontitis. *Actinobacillus actinomycetemcomitans* may be toxic to polymorphs in the gingival crevice and it is known that defective polymorph action in the gingival crevice exacerbates periodontal disease. Both organisms appear to promote destruction of fibroblasts and the activity of osteoclasts.

FURTHER READING

Dolby A.E., Walker D.M. & Matthews N (1981) *Introduction to Oral Immunology*. London, Edward Arnold.

Lehner T. & Cimasoni G. (1980) *The Borderland between Caries and Periodontal Disease II*. London, Academic Press.

Loesche W.J., Syed S.A., Laughan B.E. & Stoll J. (1982) The bacteriology of acute necrotising ulcerative gingivitis. *Journal of Periodontology*, **53**, 223–30.

Marsh P. (1979) *Oral Microbiology*. Walton-on-Thames, Nelson.

Newman M.G. & Sims T.N. (1979) The predominant culturable microbiota of the periodontal abscess. *Journal of Periodontology* **50**, 350–54.

Roitt I.M. & Lehner T. (1983) *Immunology of Oral Diseases, 2nd Edition*. Oxford, Blackwell Scientific Publications.

Schroeder H.E. & Attstrom R. (1980) Pocket formation: a hypothesis. *In* Lehner T. & Cimasoni, G. (See above).

Silverstone L.M., Johnson N.W., Hardie J.M. & Williams R.A.D. (1981) *Dental Caries, Aetiology, Pathology and Prevention*. London, MacMillan.

CHAPTER 15

Infections of the Mouth and Perioral Tissues

Dental caries and periodontal disease are the most common oral diseases in which microorganisms play an important part. Many other infections are found in the mouth and associated tissues and these may be caused by bacteria, viruses or fungi. Post-operative and other infections related to oral surgery may also be encountered.

Signs of infection. These include ulceration of the mucosae, swellings, discharging sinuses, red or white patches on the mucosae and induration of soft tissue. Symptoms include pain, especially on swallowing and

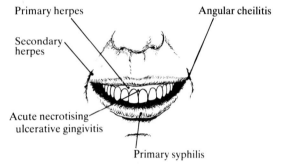

FIG. 15.2. Microbial infections of the mouth and perioral tissues.

there may be a raised temperature, malaise and lymphadenopathy. A number of infections, especially those caused by viruses, may be systemic but have oral manifestations.

Although some infections are restricted to particular sites in the mouth many microorganisms can cause lesions on the mucosae at any site. Figs. 15.1, 15.2 and 15.3 illustrate the sites at which particular microorganisms are most likely to cause infection and Table 15.1 lists the pathogens of the oral cavity and their association with the infections that will be covered in this chapter.

SURGICAL INFECTIONS AND INFECTIONS RELATED TO THE HARD TISSUES

Ludwig's angina

This describes a rapidly developing cellulitis that spreads above and below the mylohyoid. It results

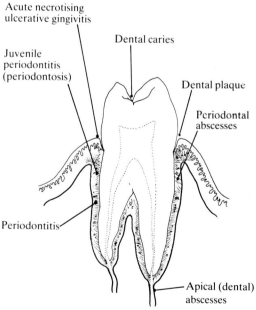

FIG. 15.1. Microbial infections of the teeth and related tissues.

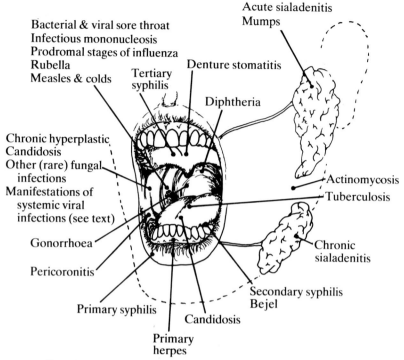

FIG. 15.3. Microbial infections of the mouth, throat and salivary glands.

from infection, usually from a dental abscess spreading posteriorly into the tissue spaces. There is marked fever and oedema of the pharynx and larynx may result in death from asphyxiation. Although a number of different bacteria have been isolated from fluid drained from the infected tissues recent reports stress the importance of anaerobic bacteria especially *Bacteroides melaninogenicus* and *gingivalis*. Treatment relies on maintaining the airway, draining fluid and giving vigorous antibiotic therapy which inevitably has to be 'blind'. If any collected fluid is analysed by gas-liquid chromatography the presence of anaerobes can be established quickly. Because of the probability of an anaerobic aetiology many clinicians include metronidazole in the spectrum of antibiotics.

Pericoronitis

This is an inflammation of the tissues surrounding a mandibular third molar that is partially erupted. The bacterial component of the condition is usually the result of multiplication of organisms in this area of stagnation resulting from the plentiful supply of nutrients. In such a reduced environment *Bacteroides melaninogenicus* and *gingivalis* are dominant.

Mechanical cleansing is often necessary prior to surgical removal of the impacted tooth. When pyrexia or lymphadenopathy is present an antibiotic, preferably penicillin, should be prescribed although metronidazole has been found to be just as successful as penicillin, underlining the probable role of anaerobes in the pathogenesis of the lesion.

Infected surgical wounds

Such infections are not common after intra-oral surgery despite the large number of bacteria that surround the wound edges. Facial incisions are more commonly infected than wounds in the mouth and staphylococci are the commonest causes of such infections. Oral streptococci, staphylococci and anaerobes such as *Bacteroides* spp and anaerobic cocci cause wound infection in the mouth.

Drainage is usually required and antibiotics may be given for cases in which there is pyrexia.

Bite wounds

Infection from the mouth can occur in bite wounds. Although human bites are often trivial and can be simply cleansed a more penetrating wound will

TABLE 15.1. Infections of the mouth.

Infection	Related or causative organism
DENTAL CARIES	*Streptococcus mutans,*? other bacteria Chap. 14)
PERIODONTAL DISEASES	*Bacteroides* spp, *Actinomyces* spp, *Capnocytophaga* spp, *Actinobacillus actinomycetemcomitans* and other organisms (Chap. 14)
SURGICAL INFECTIONS AND INFECTIONS RELATED TO HARD TISSUES	
Dry socket	Various organisms including actinomycetes. (probably none causative) (Chap. 18).
Dental abscess	Oral streptococci and many oral anaerobes (Chap. 14).
Osteomyelitis	*Staphylococcus aureus* (Chap. 18) is the most common but other bacteria may be involved.
Ludwig's angina	Oral anaerobes; beta-haemolytic streptococci
Pericoronitis	Oral anaerobes especially *Bacteroides melaninogenicus* and *gingivalis*
Surgical infected wounds	Oral streptococci, *Staphylococcus aureus, Bacteroides* spp.
BACTERIAL INFECTIONS OF THE ORAL SOFT TISSUES	
Acute	
Streptococcal stomatitis and streptococcal sore throat	Beta-haemolytic streptococci (mostly Lancefield's Group A) (Chap 16).
Diphtheria	*Corynebacterium diphtheriae* (Chap. 16)
Acute necrotising ulcerative gingivitis and Vincent's angina	Fuso-spirochaetal organisms, *Bacteroides melaninogenicus* and *gingivalis* (Chap. 14).
Gonorrhoea	*Neisseria gonorrhoeae*
Primary syphilis	*Treponema pallidum*
Acute sialadenitis	*Staphylococcus aureus*, beta-haemolytic streptococci
Chronic	
Actinomycosis	*Actinomyces israelii*
Cancrum oris (noma)	Fuso-spirochaetal organisms and *Bacteroides* spp.
Secondary and tertiary syphilis, Bejel	*Treponema pallidum*
Tuberculosis	*Mycobacterium tuberculosis*
Leprosy	*Mycobacterium leprae*
Chronic sialadenitis	Oral streptococci and *Haemophilus influenzae*
VIRAL INFECTIONS OF THE ORAL SOFT TISSUES	
Local	
Herpetic stomatitis and cold sores	Herpes simplex virus
'Shingles' or herpes zoster	Varicella-zoster virus
Sore throat	Adenovirus (Chap. 16)
Herpangina	Coxsackie A virus
As manifestations of systemic infection	
Measles	Measles virus
Mumps	Mumps virus
Chickenpox	Varicella-zoster virus
Molluscum contagiosum	Molluscum virus
Hand, foot and mouth disease	Coxsackie A virus
Glandular fever	
Burkitt's lymphoma	Epstein-Barr virus
Rabies	Rhabdovirus
FUNGAL INFECTIONS OF THE SOFT TISSUES	
Candidosis	*Candida albicans*
Histoplasmosis	*Histoplasma capsulatum*
South American blastomycosis	*Paracoccidioides brasiliensis*
Coccidioidomycosis	*Coccidioides immitis*
Sporotrichosis	*Sporotrichum schenkii*
MISCELLANEOUS CONDITIONS IN WHICH MICROORGANISMS MAY BE INVOLVED	
Behçet's and Reiter's syndromes	Chlamydia or Mycoplasma
Erythema multiforme	Mycoplasma
Stevens-Johnson syndrome	
Mucocutaneous lymph-node syndrome (Kawasaki disease)	Epstein-Barr virus and Rickettsiae (possibly of canine origin)

implant the bacteria of dental plaque deeper in the tissues and quite severe infection may result. Streptococci, anaerobic cocci and *Bacteroides* spp are the most common pathogens. Animal bites may implant other organisms, for example *Pasteurella multocida* (a Gram-negative aerobic coccobacillus) from dogs and cats which can cause a brisk inflammatory response. The organisms are often isolated in virtually pure culture. Dogs may develop chronic periodontal disease and their bites can also implant anaerobes.

BACTERIAL INFECTIONS OF THE SOFT TISSUES

Acute

Streptococcal stomatitis

This has been described as a painful red lesion developing usually on the hard palate from which beta-haemolytic streptococci, usually of Lancefield's group A, are isolated in large numbers. There is some dispute as to the existence of this condition as a separate entity from peritonsillar abscesses or streptococcal sore throat (Chap. 16). Recent reports have indicated that in the absence of beta-haemolytic streptococci in the throat isolation from lesions on the palate can be made. A rise in the antistreptolysin O titre indicates a true infection. In the absence of other infected sites in the pharynx streptococcal stomatitis is rare. Treatment with penicillin is advised.

Vincent's angina

Caused by the organisms of acute necrotising ulcerative gingivitis, spread is to the tonsils and infection is caused in the tonsillar crypts. Treatment is with metronidazole or penicillin.

Gonorrhoea

In this venereal disease caused by *Neisseria gonorrhoeae* (Chap. 20) oral infection is increasingly recognised. Presentation may vary from severe ulceration and erythema of the soft palate, buccal mucosa and gingivae to a transient and mild pharyngitis with only a diffuse reddening of the soft palate. The organisms can be seen as intracellular Gram-negative diplococci in a smear of pus from a lesion. They must, however, be cultured and their identity confirmed by carbohydrate fermentation reactions. Fluorescent antibody stains are helpful but cross-reactions with commensal species of *Branhamella* and *Neisseria* in the throat has been reported. The possibility of the presence of genital lesions should prompt referral to a venereologist who will normally treat and institute contact-tracing. An increasing number of penicillin-resistant strains have been reported necessitating the use of antibiotics such as spectinomycin or cefuroxime.

Primary syphilis

Caused by *Treponema pallidum* this is venereally acquired but oral as well as genital primary lesions have been reported. The primary lesion or chancre may be seen on the lip, tongue, buccal mucosa or palate. A history of orogenital contact may prompt the diagnosis but suspicious lesions should be handled carefully as they are infectious. The diagnosis can only be confirmed serologically (Chap. 20). Referral to a venereologist for contact-tracing is the accepted course of action. Treatment is usually with penicillin.

Acute sialadenitis

This is generally caused by viruses (see below) although *Staphylococcus aureus* and beta-haemolytic streptococci can also produce this painful infection of the salivary glands. The parotid gland is most frequently affected and the organism can be cultured from pus that emanates from the duct when the gland is palpated. Penicillin is the treatment of choice for infection with beta-haemolytic streptococci but because most strains of *Staphylococcus aureus* produce penicillinase anitbiotics such as flucloxacillin, erythromycin or a cephalosporin should be used. Surgical drainage of pus may also be required.

Chronic

Actinomycosis

Caused by *Actinomyces israelii* this is an endogenous infection. The lesions usually occur in the mandible and the soft tissues covering it and sometimes there is a recent history of surgery or tooth extraction in the vicinity. There is a thickening of the mandible and a periostitis. Single or multiple sinuses discharge generally through facial skin (Plates 10 & 11). The discharge from these sinuses is often blood-stained but if collected and allowed to stand in a glass bottle small yellow particles will settle out at the bottom. These so-called 'sulphur granules' are collections of the branching actinomycete (Plate 12). Diagnosis can be made on the clinical appearance together with microscopic examination of a sulphur granule. The organisms, however, can be cultured in an anaerobic jar and identification confirmed by carbohydrate fermentation tests or with specific fluorescent antibody. Human actinomycosis resembles the condition in cattle known as 'lumpy jaw' which is caused by *Actinomyces bovis*. Occasionally other organisms can be isolated together with *Actinomyces israelii* from lesions of human actinomycosis such as *Actinobacillus actinomycetemcomitans* (Chap. 14). Treatment of actinomycosis is often protracted. Surgical drainage of any pus that can drain through the hard tissues is beneficial. Penicillin or erythromycin may be used but treatment may be required for eight weeks or more.

Cancrum oris (Noma)

This is a condition found almost exclusively in tropical Africa and Asia. The often devastating necrotising and ulcerative lesions produce a sloughing of much of the cheek and lip with exposure of the bone and teeth. It is thought that the lesion develops from acute necrotising ulcerative gingivitis and is thus associated with the fuso-spirochaetal organisms and *Bacteroides* spp. It is not clear why the infection becomes much more rampant among the African and Asian races of the tropics than among negroes of the U.S.A. or the white races, although malnutrition may account for this. A concurrent infection such as measles may also be a factor; measles is known to be much more serious disease in tropical areas than in temperature zones. Treatment with metronidazole or penicillin with supportive nutritional supplementation is necessary and plastic surgery may also be required.

Secondary and tertiary syphilis

Both stages of the disease show oral signs. In secondary syphilis snail track ulcers and mucous patches can be seen. These lesions are highly infective and should be touched only with gloved hands. Gummata and leukoplakia are characteristic of tertiary syphilis and these frequently occur in the mouth, especially on the hard palate. If diagnosis of the primary chancre has been missed then the patient presenting with lesions resembling secondary syphilis should be referred to a venereologist. Serological tests will confirm the diagnosis. Penicillin can be used for treating syphilis at the secondary stage but there is no active infection present in tertiary syphilis so antibiotics are useless.

Bejel

This is a form of endemic syphilis found in the Middle East and Balkans. Primary infection is usually oral; genital lesions are uncommon. The disease usually starts in childhood and progresses more slowly than the classical venereal syphilis. Treatment with penicillin in the early stages is curative. Endemic syphilis seen among Greenland eskimoes is not Bejel but is characteristic of the venereal disease, with genital primary lesions and oral secondary, tertiary and congenital lesions.

Tuberculosis

Once a common cause of oral ulceration this is associated with patients with active pulmonary tuberculosis. Tuberculous oral ulceration is therefore seen in poorer countries where pulmonary disease is still common. An irregularly shaped ulcer with a grey slough is characteristic of the lesion. Diagnosis is often difficult because Ziehl-Neelsen-stained smears rarely show *Mycobacterium tuberculosis* in the lesions. The presence of active pulmonary tuberculosis increases suspicion but diagnosis is usually made only after biopsy of a chronic ulcer. Cases should be referred to a chest physician who will start antituberculous therapy. It is important that dental personnel in close contract with a patient with oral or active pulmonary tuberculosis should receive appropriate prophylaxis.

Leprosy

Mycobacterium leprae is the cause of this disease, nowadays rarely seen outside the tropics. Nodules appear on the oral mucosae in lepromatous leprosy and these often ulcerate and become scarred. Leprosy bacilli cannot be cultured in artificial media but they can be seen in stained smears of nodules of lepromatous leprosy. Nodules, often quite disfiguring, also occur on the facial skin.

Chronic sialadenitis

This occurs usually in the submandibular gland but also in the parotid. Oral streptococci and *Haemophilus influenzae* are the most frequent isolates. The damaged gland has impaired drainage and because of fluid accumulation and stasis bacteria invade and multiply. Antibiotics are often only of limited value but may be helpful at times. Surgical excision of any calculus or constriction of the duct is required.

VIRAL INFECTIONS OF THE ORAL SOFT TISSUES

Local

Herpetic stomatitis

This is caused by the DNA virus herpes simplex, usually type 1.

The primary infection. Is generally seen in children and follows about one week after exposure to the virus. It presents as an acute gingivostomatitis (Fig.

ganglion. Virus can no longer be detected in saliva or on the mucosae.

Secondary infection. This usually manifests as 'cold sores' (Fig. 15.5). The virus passes down the sensory nerve from cell to cell thus avoiding the neutralising effect of antibody. Reactivation of the virus is usually a result of an upper respiratory tract infection. The virus produces vesicular lesions at the mucocutaneous junctions around lips and nostrils. These lesions usually appear unilaterally and are confined to the distribution of either the maxillary or the mandibular divisions of the trigeminal nerve. Although

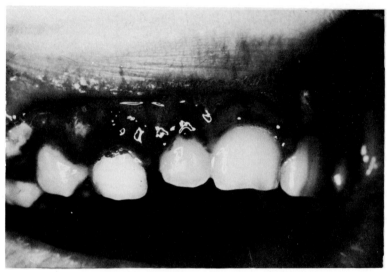

FIG. 15.4. Acute herpetic gingivostomatitis.

15.4) somewhat similar to acute necrotising ulcerative gingivitis but without loss of inter-dental papillae. There are large numbers of vesicles that cover the lips, gingivae, ventral aspect of the tongue and other oral mucosal surfaces. These vesicles rapidly ulcerate and the coallescing ulcers may cover large areas of mucosa. The patient is often febrile and there is a regional lymphadenopathy. The condition subsides in about 10 days and specific antibody levels rise two to three weeks after the onset. Surveys of antibody titres to herpes simplex show that most of the adult population have antibody (97 per cent) but as fewer cases of primary herpetic gingivostomatitis are seen than would be expected, clearly many subclinical primary infections occur.

Latent period. After the primary infection subsides the virus migrates along the sensory fibres of the trigeminal nerve and lies latent in the trigeminal

the lesions fade after about one week the virus is not eliminated and returns to its latent state in the trigeminal ganglion. Secondary infection is usually trivial but it can be severe in immunosuppressed patients.

Other manifestations of herpes simplex infection. These include herpetic whitlow where the finger becomes infected with the virus, producing a painful erythematous lesion (Fig. 15.5). It is easily contracted by a dentist examining herpetic lesions with ungloved hands. Herpetic keratitis is a recurrent infection of the eye with ulceration and sometimes scarring of the cornea (Ch. 21).

Treatment of oral herpes infections usually entails supportive therapy, especially adequate fluid and nutritional intake in young children with primary infection. Drugs are rarely used. Idoxuridine has not been especially helpful in speeding recovery from

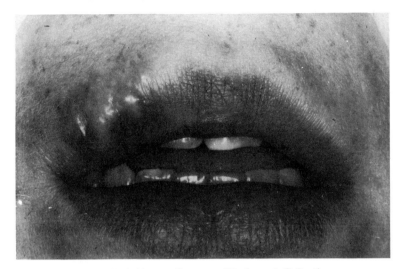

FIG. 15.5. Cold sores. Courtesy of Professor J. C. Southam.

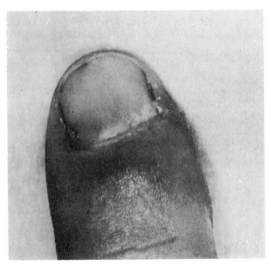

FIG. 15.6. Herpetic whitlow.

primary or secondary infection. Immunosuppressed patients may be severely affected and for these idoxuridine or acyclovir may be useful.

'Shingles' or Herpes zoster

This is caused by a herpes virus Varicella-zoster. The primary infection is chickenpox but the recurrent infection is usually restricted to the distribution on the skin of one sensory nerve. Reactivation of the virus usually occurs in adulthood many years after the primary infection of childhood chickenpox. The lesions consist of a crop of vesicular eruptions often distributed on the thorax, but the trigeminal nerve can be involved, usually the ophthalmic division. Sensory (tympanic) branches of the facial nerve may be affected (Ramsay-Hunt syndrome). Vesicles then appear on the forehead and eyelids. Less commonly the maxillary or mandibular division of the nerve may be involved and therefore the oral mucosae affected. Idoxuridine if applied promptly to early eruptions speeds up their resolution often preventing their full development. Severe cases may require acyclovir.

Herpangina

This is characterised by a crop of tiny ulcers on the oral mucosae that coallesce and fade after about one week. Lesions are seen on the soft palate and the patient complains of a sore throat. Coxsackie A virus (usually Type 4) is the cause of this condition. Chlorhexidine gluconate or chlortetracycline mouth rinses may prevent bacterial multiplication at the base of the ulcers and speed up healing of the lesions.

As manifestations of systemic infection

Measles

This is a childhood fever that starts with a prodromal respiratory illness. During this period small white spots can be seen on the buccal mucosae opposite the molar teeth. These Koplik's spots are surrounded by erythema and may number from a few to several hundred. Their appearance is transitory and as the generalised signs of measles appear—maculopapular rash and fever—so the Koplik's spots subside. Measles confers life-long immunity on the host.

In tropical countries where malnutrition is common measles can be a devastating disease. The oral lesions become ulcerated, often severely, and some patients develop cancrum oris probably from a concurrent acute necrotising ulcerative gingivitis.

Mumps

Although this is the most common cause of acute parotitis the submandibular glands can also become affected. The mumps virus causes a generalised infection and glandular tissue and neural tissues are particularly affected. Other viruses can cause parotitis including Coxsackie A, parainfluenza and ECHO viruses. Treatment consists of supportive therapy; antiviral drugs are not administered. Complications in the salivary gland are not common but adults may develop pancreatitis and orchitis.

Chickenpox

The childhood illness is caused by the herpes virus zoster. The characteristic rash of vesicles may affect the oral mucosae but these vesicles are usually asymptomatic and heal rapidly. The virus becomes latent after infection and although there is lasting immunity to chickenpox the host remains susceptible to zoster in later life.

Molluscum contagiosum

Caused by a pox virus of the same name this is characterised by nodular lesions resembling warts, mainly seen on the skin of the trunk or axilla, although facial skin and oral mucous membranes can be affected. The disease is most common in children and lasts for a few months. There is no specific treatment but secondary infection of oral lesions often occurs and chlorhexidine mouth rinses may help prevent these.

Hand, foot and mouth disease

This is caused by Coxsackie A virus, usually types 16, 5 and 10 and also by enterovirus 71. This disease is not to be confused with foot and mouth disease, an infection of cattle that has only very rarely been transmitted to man through the handling of heavily infected carcases. The oral component of hand, foot and mouth disease consists of a crop of painful ulcers resembling those of herpangina that are usually located on the soft palate. Vesicles also appear on the palms of the hands and soles of the feet. Children are most commonly affected but adult infection is not rare. The infection often occurs in small localised outbreaks.

Glandular fever

The Epstein–Barr virus (EBV) another member of the herpesvirus group, causes this. Young adults are characteristically affected. There is general malaise, fatigue, fever and lymphadenopathy which may be generalised or localised to the head and neck. There is often a sore throat and the tonsils may be inflamed. Petechial haemorrhages are sometimes seen on the soft palate and oral ulceration of the palate is common. Sometimes there is a whitish exudate covering the soft palate.

Blood films show large atypical lymphocytes and there is a lymphocytosis. Diagnosis is on the basis of the Paul–Bunnell test for the presence of heterophil antibody or the detection of specific IgM antibody to the virus immunofluorescence. If ampicillin is given for the sore throat a sensitivity reaction frequently occurs even in patients not normally hypersensitive to the penicillins. Treatment is supportive but recent reports have suggested that metronidazole may speed up resolution of the anginose form of the disease in which there are petechial haemorrhages on the palate and tonsils. Anginose forms of infectious mononucleosis may be caused by a mixed infection of glandular fever with a superimposed Vincent's angina and so the reduction of anaerobes in the inflamed tissues speeds up recovery. The oral lesions and lymphadenopathy generally resolve in three weeks.

Other manifestations of EBV infection. Another manifestation of EBV infection is seen in Burkitt's lymphoma in which the virus is thought to play an important role in the development of the neoplasm. Burkitt's lymphoma is the commonest neoplasm seen in children in parts of Africa. Lesions are present in the jaws or close to the orbit. Antibody to EBV is found in all cases of Burkitt's lymphoma and the virus has been isolated from tumour tissue in many cases. Other factors, as yet unknown, are presumably involved in initiating a lymphoma after infection with EBV in children in tropical Africa. Although EBV infection outside this part of the world is manifested as glandular fever there is now some evidence linking the virus to nasopharyngeal carcinoma in which antibodies to EBV are again invariably found.

Other viral diseases

Several may occur in the mouth. In particular the lesions termed herpetiform ulceration resemble those seen in genuine viral infections of the oral mucosae. So far, however, no virus has yet been identified. Rabies is a viral disease transmitted to man from the bite of an infected animal, for example dogs and foxes. The virus is present in the saliva of the animal and passes along nerves to the brain where the resulting encephalitis is almost invariably fatal. Although there are no oral lesions the saliva of human cases of rabies is loaded with virus particles.

FUNGAL INFECTIONS OF THE SOFT TISSUES

Candidosis (candidiasis, moniliasis)

This is caused by the yeast *Candida albicans*. Similar lesions in the mouth may be caused by other species of candida such as *Candida tropicalis* and also by *Torulopsis glabrata*.

Oral candidosis can present in a number of ways (Table 15.2).

Acute pseudomembraneous candidosis (Fig. 15.7). This occurs in infancy, old age and in debilitated patients. This form of candidosis only appears when host defence mechanisms are compromised, or, in the case of young babies, not yet established. Any of the mucosal surfaces of the mouth may be covered in white plaques or pseudomembranes. These can easily be rubbed off but they mostly leave an area of erythema or bleeding. The diagnosis can be confirmed by microscopic examination of the white

TABLE 15.2. Manifestations of candidosis in the mouth.

ACUTE
  Pseudomembranous
    —Oral thrush
  Atrophic
    —Antibiotic sore mouth
CHRONIC
  Atrophic
    — (1) Denture stomatitis
    — (2) Angular cheilitis
  Hyperplastic
    — (1) Confined to mouth
    — (2) Mucocutaneous
    — (3) Mucocutaneous but associated with endocrine abnormalities

pseudomembrane. Pseudohyphae and yeasts that are Gram-positive will be seen. They also readily take up the periodic-acid-Schiff stain (Fig 15.8). One of the anti-candidal drugs such as amphotericin or nystatin is used in treatment. These should be sucked in order to achieve a topical action. It is vital that the underlying predisposition be corrected and referral to a general physician may be required. Common predisposing factors include iron deficiency, diabetes and drug therapy with immunosuppressives, steroids or broad-spectrum antibiotics.

Acute atrophic candidosis. Broad spectrum antibiotics such as tetracyline and ampicillin are responsible for this infection. They reduce the normal flora

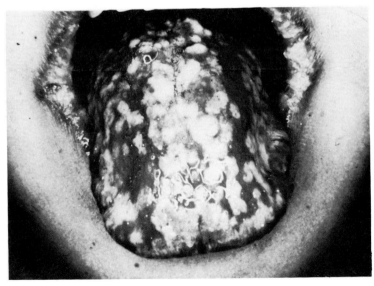

FIG. 15.7. Acute pseudomembranous candidosis.

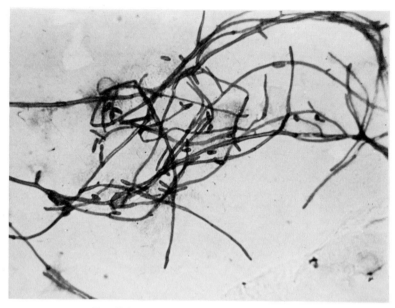

FIG. 15.8. Pseudomycelium of *Candida albicans*

drastically and the vacant sites on the epithelium become colonised with yeasts. This overgrowth of yeasts produces atrophic and inflamed mucosae. Yeasts can generally be grown on culture though Gram-stained smears are frequently negative, probably because of the difficulty in obtaining a good scraping of atrophic mucosae. Treatment consists of stopping the antibiotic or changing to one with a narrower spectrum to allow the normal flora to return. Occasionally antifungal drugs are required.

Chronic atrophic candidosis. Occurring under the fitting surface of dentures, usually confined to the palate, this is the most common manifestation of oral candidosis. The palate appears red, petechiae are sometimes seen and in long-standing cases papillary hyperplasia occurs in the vault of the palate (Fig 15.9) *Candida* multiplies and invades the tissues, largely because the normal oral flora is reduced in the altered conditions under the denture. If dentures are removed for part of every 24-hour day, for example at

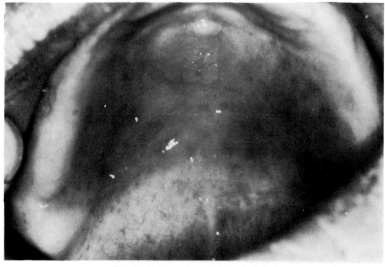

FIG. 15.9. Chronic atrophic candidosis.

night the condition is seen much less frequently. Not only does the palate become invaded but the acrylic denture base is heavily colonised by the organism and this may form the reservoir for repeated infection. There is no evidence for allergy to acrylic or other denture material having any part to play in the aetiology of this condition. Hyphae and yeast forms can be seen on Gram- or periodic acid-Schiff-stained smears. Culture will yield large numbers of the organism. There seems to be little doubt that *Candida albicans* can cause denture stomatitis as reversion to a normal flora by removing dentures causes a reduction in the numbers of yeasts present and a resolution of the erythema. Treatment with anti-candidal drugs may often have to be prolonged. Recurrence is common. Soaking the denture in chlorhexidine helps reduce the numbers of yeasts residing on the acrylic denture that could establish re-infection.

Angular cheilitis. This occurs mainly in edentulous patients who have a reduction in the vertical height of their face due to long term wearing of dentures. Often an associated denture stomatitis is seen. Saliva moistens the commissures and the macerated skin soon becomes infected with yeasts. Increasing the vertical dimension of the face and construction of new dentures will help remove this condition. Initially anti-candidal drugs in ointment bases may promote healing.

Angular cheilitis may occur in dentate patients. *Staphylococcus aureus* is a common finding from such lesions alone or with *Candida albicans*. A few cases are infected with beta-haemolytic streptococci. Treatment may involve antibiotic ointments. Topical penicillins are not advised because of the dangers of hypersensitivity. Often chlorhexidine gel is adequate.

Chronic hyperplastic candidosis. Sometimes termed 'candida leucoplakia', the lesions in this condition are white, firmly adherent and often raised. Any part of the mucosae may be affected but the buccal mucosa, and tongue are the commonest sites. The lesion which may be an isolated one in the mouth may become ulcerated and should be regarded as potentially premalignant. Treatments vary from surgical excision of small or suspicious lesions to the administration of anti-candidal drugs. Miconazole and other imidazoles are abdorbed from the gastrointestinal tract and salivary levels remain high. The topical and systemic effect gained with these drugs may be beneficial in treating chronic hyperplastic candidosis compared with amphotericin or nystatin.

Chronic mucocutaneous candidosis may also affect other mucous surfaces, notably the vagina. Skin and especially nail beds may be involved. Clearly factors other than candidal infection are implicated in such cases and more remains to be discovered about the immunological and genetic aspects of this disease. One association is recognised — that of hypoparathyroidism with chronic mucocutaneous candidosis, and some of these rare cases are known to have inherited the condition as an autosomal recessive trait.

Histoplasmosis

Caused by the dimorphic fungus *Histoplasma capsulatum* from contaminated soil, this may be a serious, often fatal, generalised disease or a mild asymptomatic pulmonary infection. In parts of the USA asymptomatic infection is common. There may be granulomas of the skin, mouth and pharynx and ulceration of the oral mucosae. Oral lesions also occur in the usually fatal disseminated disease. Treatment with imidazoles or amphotericin may be effective.

South American blastomycosis

This is caused by the dimorphic fungus *Paracoccidioides brasiliensis* and infection is largely confined to Brazil where it is not uncommon. The initial lesions are usually oral with granulomatous ulcers on any oral surface. The fungus spreads by the lymphatics and may affect almost any tissue of the body. Scraping the ulcer bed will yield the fungus on culture.

Coccidioidomycosis

Another fungal infection of the Americas, this occurs largely in California and Central America. The fungus, *Coccidioides immitis* may cause fatal disseminated disease but a self-limiting disease is more common. This latter condition may be a mild pulmonary infection or may present either as oral ulceration or crusting, ulcerative or nodular lesions on the face. Treatment with anti-fungal drugs is usually only required for progressive disease.

Sporotrichosis

A common mycosis in Central America this is also seen in Europe the U.S.A. It is caused by *Sporotrichum schenkii* In some forms of this rather varied disease oral ulceration occurs and granulomatous lesions resembling actinomycosis may be seen on facial skin. Anti-fungal drugs are effective in treating these lesions.

MISCELLANEOUS CONDITIONS IN WHICH MICROORGANISMS MAY CONTRIBUTE TO THE AETIOLOGY

Behçet's and Reiter's syndromes

Ulceration of the oral mucosae, genital mucosae, uveitis and arthritis are features common to both syndromes although not all features will be seen in any one patient. Behçet's Syndrome may also be characterised by skin, vascular and neurological disorders. There have been several attempts to associate these syndromes with infective agents but none of the evidence is conclusive. *Chlamydia* and *Mycoplasma* spp have, however, been associated with Reiter's syndrome. There are strong associations between tissue type as determined by the HLA (human leucocyte antigen) system and the presence of these disorders. Reiter's syndrome is associated with type HLA-B27 and Behçet's syndrome with HLA-B5, HLA-B12 and HLA-B27. Nevertheless, only a small proportion of patients possessing these HLA types develop the disease.

Erythema multiforme and Stevens-Johnson syndrome

The oral lesions of these conditions often resemble a severe viral infection with large coallescing ulcers of lips and mucosae. Ocular, genital and skin lesions are also commonly seen. A maculopapular skin eruption and mucosal lesions of two orifices are required to qualify for the term 'Stevens-Johnson Syndrome'. The less severe forms of the disease are termed erythma multiforme. Microbial associations have often been reported, particularly with *Mycoplasma pneumoniae*. Strong links with recent drug therapy have been reported especially with antimicrobials such as sulphonamides and contrimoxazole.

Mucocutaneous lymph-node syndrome (Kawasaki disease)

This condition which generally affects children has several features in common with the other mucocutaneous syndromes. There is fever, a rash on the skin and inflammation of the oral mucosa, tongue and conjunctiva. There is cervical lymphadenopathy and several systemic disturbances have been reported. Rickettsiae of canine origin have been associated with this disease in Japan and a deranged immune response to Epstein-Barr virus has also been reported.

FURTHER READING

Burnett G.W. & Schuster G.S. (1978) *Oral Microbiology and Infectious Disease*, Student Edition Baltimore, Williams & Wilkins.

Dolby A.E., Walker D.M. & Matthews N. (1981) *Introduction to Oral Immunology*, London, Edward Arnold.

Gayford J.J. & Haskell R. (1979) *Clinical Oral Medicine*, 2nd Edition. Bristol, John Wright.

Killey H.C., Seward G.R. & Kay L.W. (1975) *An Outline of Oral Surgery*. Part 1 Revised Reprint. Bristol, John Wright.

Tyldesley W.R. (1981) *Oral Medicine*. Oxford, Oxford University Press.

CHAPTER 16

Infections of the Respiratory Tract

The respiratory tract is the most common site of infections in man and although these are mostly mild and associated with the cold, damp winter months they can nevertheless be very serious, particularly in the old and young and in the compromised patient and can occur throughout the year.

Respiratory infections may be acute or chronic and can be caused by several different forms of microorganisms such as bacteria, viruses, rickettsiae, chlamydiae, mycoplasmas and fungi. For convenience they are commmonly described as upper and lower respiratory tract infections although some infectious agents, notably viruses, affect both areas simultaneously.

Normal flora

Although the lower respiratory tract in health is sterile, several species of organisms colonise the upper respiratory tract, particularly the nose and throat. These are predominantly aerobes and include species of staphylococci, streptococci including pneumococci, corynebacteria, *Haemophilus* and neisseriae.

Defences against infection (Table 16.1).

Potential pathogens (Fig. 16.1).

The common cold

Parainfluenza viruses, respiratory syncytial viruses (RSV), rhinoviruses, corona, coxsackie and Echo viruses are the most frequent causes of the common cold.

TABLE 16.1. Defences against infection in the respiratory tract.

The vibrissae of the nose
Bronchoconstriction
The cough reflex
Mucus glands and goblet cells
Action of cilia
Non-specific mucosal factors (alpha-antitrypsin, lactoferrin and lysozyme)
Lymphatics of the bronchi and bronchioles
The alveolar macrophage system
Local humoral mucosal antibody (secretory IgA)
Local cell-mediated immunity

Parainfluenza viruses are also associated with croup in infants. There are four such viruses. They can be isolated from mouth washings and throat swabs and are grown in monkey kidney cell lines. Complement fixation tests are also used in diagnosis.

RSV causes the common cold in older children but it is also responsible for severe attacks of bronchiolitis and pneumonia in infants, particularly in the winter months. RSV is a paramyxovirus which is isolated from mouth washings and nasal secretions; HEp 2 and monkey kidney cells are inoculated and cytopathic effects (CPE) looked for. Complement fixation tests and direct immunofluorescence are helpful in establishing the diagnosis.

Rhinoviruses (picornaviruses) comprise many different serotypes and are isolated from nasal secretions and mouth washings. There are two groups. 'M' rhinoviruses grow only in monkey tissue culture with CPE, and 'H' rhinoviruses grow only in human embryo tissue with CPE.

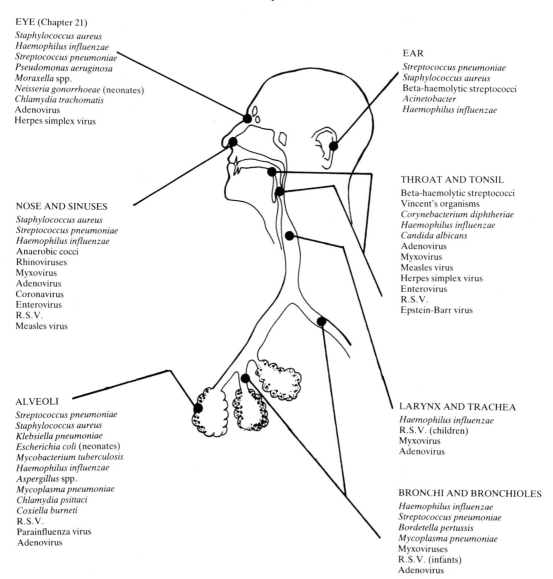

EYE (Chapter 21)
Staphylococcus aureus
Haemophilus influenzae
Streptococcus pneumoniae
Pseudomonas aeruginosa
Moraxella spp.
Neisseria gonorrhoeae (neonates)
Chlamydia trachomatis
Adenovirus
Herpes simplex virus

EAR
Streptococcus pneumoniae
Staphylococcus aureus
Beta-haemolytic streptococci
Acinetobacter
Haemophilus influenzae

NOSE AND SINUSES
Staphylococcus aureus
Streptococcus pneumoniae
Haemophilus influenzae
Anaerobic cocci
Rhinoviruses
Myxovirus
Adenovirus
Coronavirus
Enterovirus
R.S.V.
Measles virus

THROAT AND TONSIL
Beta-haemolytic streptococci
Vincent's organisms
Corynebacterium diphtheriae
Haemophilus influenzae
Candida albicans
Adenovirus
Myxovirus
Measles virus
Herpes simplex virus
Enterovirus
R.S.V.
Epstein-Barr virus

ALVEOLI
Streptococcus pneumoniae
Staphylococcus aureus
Klebsiella pneumoniae
Escherichia coli (neonates)
Mycobacterium tuberculosis
Haemophilus influenzae
Aspergillus spp.
Mycoplasma pneumoniae
Chlamydia psittaci
Coxiella burneti
R.S.V.
Parainfluenza virus
Adenovirus

LARYNX AND TRACHEA
Haemophilus influenzae
R.S.V. (children)
Myxovirus
Adenovirus

BRONCHI AND BRONCHIOLES
Haemophilus influenzae
Streptococcus pneumoniae
Bordetella pertussis
Mycoplasma pneumoniae
Myxoviruses
R.S.V. (infants)
Adenovirus

FIG. 16.1. Potential pathogens of the respiratory tract.

Enteroviruses associated with respiratory tract infections include Coxsackie A21 (Coe virus) and echoviruese 11 and 20.

Infectious mononucleosis (glandular fever)

This acute febrile illness is caused by the Epstein-Barr (EB) virus, a member of the Herpes group.

Diagnosis. This is by the Paul-Bunnell (haemagglutination) test, by the demonstration by immunofluorescence of virus-specific IgM or a rising titre of specific IgG and by the appearance of atypical lymphocytes in the blood.

Infection of the paranasal sinuses

This can be acute or chronic and is caused by pneumococci, anaerobic cocci, *Haemophilus influenzae*, *Staphylococcus aureus* and beta-haemolytic streptococci, bacteria that colonise adjacent areas. Infection occurs in association with obstruction resulting from mucosal oedema. Inflammation of the sinuses is common in virus infections of the upper respiratory tract. Maxillary sinusitis sometimes mimics toothache in the maxillary molar teeth on the affected side.

Otitis media

Frequently otitis media is the result of direct spread of pathogens, namely pneumococci, *Haemophilus influenzae* and beta-haemolytic streptococci, from the throat via the Eustachian tube. This infection can be acute or chronic and may be caused by viruses and mycoplasmas as well as bacteria. In the young the bacteria most frequently involved are pneumococci, *Haemophilus influenzae* and beta-haemolytic streptococci, whereas in older patients *Haemophilus*

foot and mouth disease, rubella and infectious mononucleosis.

Prodromal stage of viral infection of the respiratory tract. Viruses involved in such infections include adenovirus, influenza, parainfluenza and rhino-viruses.

Diphtheria

Bacterial aetiology. Corynebacterium diphtheriae; gravis, intermedius and *mitis* are the three main biotypes.

Pathogenesis and epidemiology. Diphtheria begins as an acute inflammatory condition of the upper respiratory tract, usually the throat. A powerful

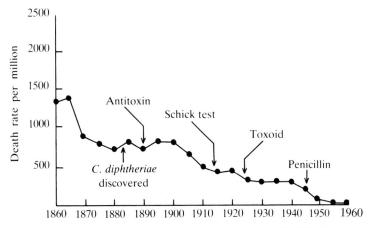

FIG. 16.2. Decline in incidence of diphtheria in the U.K., 1860–1960.

influenzae, Staphylococcus aureus, pneumococci, and in chronic cases, coliform organisms, may be responsible. There is a risk of mastoiditis in cases of untreated bacterial otitis media.

Sore throat

Infective causes of sore throat:
    (1) prodromal stage of infectious diseases.
    (2) prodromal stage of viral infection of the respiratory tract,
    (3) diphtheria,
    (4) Vincent's angina (Chap. 14), and
    (5) 'sore throat syndrome'.

Prodromal stages of infectious diseases. Several infectious diseases may cause sore throat before the appearance of rashes, vesicles or other signs, including chickenpox, measles, meningitis, hand,

exotoxin is produced which diffuses through the body affecting the myocardium, adrenal glands and nerve endings. At the site of infection the inflammatory exudate and necrotic mucosal cells form a membrane that remains adherent to the throat and this may produce respiratory obstruction. Figure 16.2 shows the pattern of the disease in the U.K. during the last century. The carriage rate in the U.K. of toxigenic corynebacteria is now negligible due to the national immunisation programme but non-toxigenic strains have been isolated from immigrant children.

Laboratory diagnosis. Selective media containing tellurite are used as well as precipitin tests and guinea pig inoculation.

Prophylaxis. In order to keep diphtheria at the present level of control active immunisation is the most important measure. It is best to give diphtheria and tetanus toxoids with pertussis vaccine (triple vaccine) in three separate doses, beginning in the third month of life; there should be an interval of six to eight weeks and four to six months between the first, second and third injections respectively. A booster dose is given at school entry, omitting the pertussis element.

Treatment. Antitoxin in addition to penicillin or erythromycin must be used.

The sore throat syndrome (STS)

Bacterial aetiology. The STS is essentially an acute pharyngitis and/or an acute tonsillitis and is caused by bacteria, viruses and mycoplasmas. The bacteria are usually the Lancefield group A beta-haemolytic streptococci, *Streptococus pyogenes*. Groups C and G and rarely F may also be involved, but other bacteria are only very rarely implicated. A bacterial sore throat implies a streptococcal sore throat, except in the compromised host in whom a variety of bacteria may produce infection. It is important to remember that only 30–40 per cent of cases of the STS are caused by streptococci; the remaining cases are most likely caused by viruses, such as adenovirus (frequently also associated with conjunctivitis), rhinovirus, influenza, enteroviruses and EB viruses, or by *Mycoplasma pneumoniae*.

Pathogenesis and epidemiology. Sore throat is very common especially in the winter months but it is uncommon in the under two-year olds and in the elderly. Its peak incidence is in the young school child who has a poorly developed level and range of antibodies. It is much less common in the older school child, adolescent and young adult. Rarely a streptococcal sore throat can be contracted from eating contaminated food or drinking contaminated milk.

Laboratory diagnosis. Swabs should be sent off quickly to the laboratory. If delay in collection or in transit is anticipated swabs should be stored in the refrigerator as this helps preserve streptococci. A sample of saliva may also be sent off in addition to the throat swab as many patients with streptococcal sore throat shed streptococci into the saliva.

Gram films of throat swabs are not helpful, although they will show up any *Candida* organisms present. Swabs should be plated on blood media and on crystal violet. The haemolysis of many beta-haemolytic streptococci is enhanced after anaerobic incubation of culture plates. A bacitracin disk can help to differentiate group A from other beta-

haemolytic streptococci (group A is mostly sensitive) but streptococcal grouping tests should be performed in doubtful cases.

STS cannot be diagnosed on clinical evidence because symptoms and signs produced by both streptococci and viruses are similar. The appearance of the throat is of little diagnostic help as non-infected throats can appear red, whereas *Streptococcus pyogenes* may be cultured from pale, normal-looking throats.

Treatment. Beta-haemolytic streptococci are universally sensitive to penicillin. Erythromycin is also a very useful drug in cases of penicillin hypersensitivity.

Acute epiglottitis: Acute laryngo-tracheo-bronchitis.

Bacterial aetiology. Although viruses may be associated with both conditions, *Haemophilus influenzae, type b,* is the important causative organism.

Pathogenesis and epidemiology. Both conditions affect infants and young children and are frequently fulminating. Acute epiglottitis in young children due to *Haemophilus influenzae* may cause acute respiratory obstruction.

Laboratory diagnosis. In both infections there is a septicaemic phase and blood culture is frequently positive. Pharyngeal swabs may also be helpful.

Treatment. Because of the severity of both infections antibiotic therapy has to be on a 'best guess' basis, and penicillin or ampicillin may be used until the laboratory confirms the diagnosis.

Influenza

Influenza is one of the major epidemic diseases and spreads rapidly from area to area. At times it becomes pandemic and sweeps throughout the entire world. Spread is by the respiratory route.

Recovery is usually complete but in a small minority of cases pneumonia may follow, either a primary influenzal pneumonia or a secondary bacterial one. Both forms are severe and death is common. Flu-like illnesses can be caused by an assortment of other respiratory tract viruses.

Types of virus: There are three types of influenza virus - A, the main cause of influenza, B associated with less severe forms of the disease and C, of low pathogenicity. They have three main antigens - 'S' or soluble antigen which is type specific; a haemagglutinin which is strain specific; and neuraminidase.

Antigenic variation: A feature of virus A strains is antigenic variation - major variation (antigenic shift) and minor variation (antigenic drift). The major form is due to the emergence of a new strain of virus containing a new haemagglutin or neuraminidase. Sometimes both can occur. Minor change is due to change in the amino acid sequence of the haemagglutinin which is protein in nature. The most important practical feature about major antigenic variation is that there is no immunity in the population to the new strain. Existing antibodies to strains formerly prevalent in the community confer no protection against the new strain which can spread through populations very rapidly, causing widespread epidemics.

Diagnosis: Mouth washings and throat swabs are used in diagnosis. Monkey kidney tissue cultures and the amniotic cavity of chick embryos are inoculated. Haemadsorption of human group O and fowl

erythrocytes occurs in positive cultures. The virus is typed by haemagglutination-inhibition tests with specific antisera. Antibody to influenza may also be detected by complement fixation and haemagglutination inhibition.

Prophylaxis: Two types of vaccine exist, live attenuated and inactivated. In general the live vaccines are more effective than the killed. The vaccine viruses must be those that circulate in the community, but as they will not protect against antigenic shift in the virus vaccines have to be constantly brought up to date. A moderate degree of protection is possible.

Whooping cough

Bacterial aetiology. Bordetella pertussis.

Pathogenesis and epidemiology. Infection is spread by direct droplet spray and in unprotected children the secondary attack rate in a family may be around 90 per cent. Whooping cough occurs in epidemic proportions every few years. It is a serious disease in

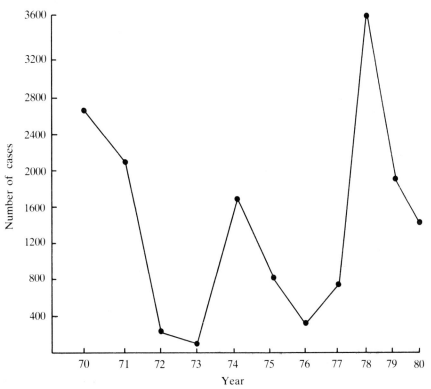

FIG. 16.3. Whooping cough in Scotland, 1970–80. Confirmed notifications. Source–Information Services Division, Common Services Agency of the Scottish Health Service.

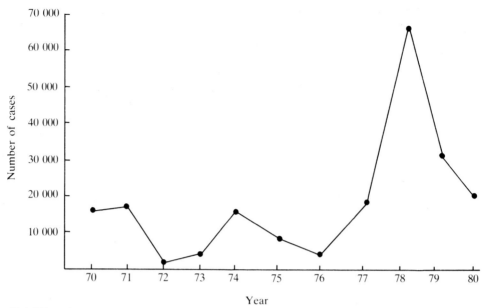

FIG. 16.4. Whooping cough in England and Wales, 1970–80. Source–Registrar General's Annual Statistical Reviews of England and Wales.

young children, especially females, and approximately 10 per cent of children under two years of age who contract the disease have to be admitted to hospital. The fatality rate in children under one year of age is 50 times higher than on one to four year olds and 100 times greater than in five to nine year olds. Immunity by infection or by immunisation is long lasting, and in so-called second attacks of whooping cough the possibility of an infection by *Bordetella parapertussis*, or by viruses (such as parainfluenza and adeno) should be considered. Figs. 16.3 and 16.4 show whooping cough rates in Scotland and England and Wales over the last few years.

Laboratory diagnosis. A pernasal swab or cough plate containing Bordet-Gengou or charcoal medium should be examined by the usual methods and a swab may also be examined by immunofluorescence. With a good technique the organisms can be isolated from almost every case in the early stage of the disease if the patient is not on antibiotics. As time progresses isolation becomes more difficult but by the end of the second week serological tests such as agglutination and complement fixation tests can be performed.

Prophylaxis. Bordetella pertussis is included in the triple vaccine. Antibiotic prophylaxis using drugs such as erythromycin has been suggested for children at risk from the infection who cannot be immunised.

Treatment. Bordetella pertussis is sensitive to many antibiotics but these do little to influence the course of the disease.

Bronchitis

Bacterial aetiology. Two organisms predominate in acute exacerbations of chronic bronchitis, *Haemophilus influenzae* and *Streptococcus pneumoniae*.

Pathogenesis and epidemiology. Chronic bronchitis is a relapsing condition, common in the U.K. Various factors are involved in addition to infection, namely smoking, previous lung damage, atmospheric pollution and cold damp weather.

Laboratory diagnosis. Sputum samples are examined although the diagnosis is easily made clinically. One of the main reasons for culture is to check on antibiograms of the probable pathogens.

Treatment. Each acute episode can be treated as it occurs or the patient can be put on a long-term course of antibiotics over the winter months. In the latter event it is mandatory to check periodically the antibiotic sensitivities of any *Haemophilus* organisms isolated. Broad-spectrum antibiotics such as tetracyclines and ampicillin are useful in this infection but treatment must depend on sensitivity test results.

Pneumonia

Bacterial aetiology. Lobar pneumonia is invariably caused by *Streptococcus pneumoniae* whereas bronchopneumonia can be caused by many pathogens.

Pathogenesis and epidemiology. The two main infective types are lobar and bronchopneumonia, although other types such as hypostatic and aspiration are described; these names refer rather to predisposing factors than to separate pathological entities.

Cross infection is the main means of production of lobar pneumonia, although infection may be caused by the pneumococci in the patient's own upper respiratory tract flora. There are over 80 pneumococcal serotypes but only a few are implicated in the majority of attacks. The pathogenesis involves invasion of the alveoli with subsequent deprivation of alveolar cells of adequate nutrition, resistance of the capsulate organisms to phagocytes and the production of one or more exotoxins, such as pneumolysin.

In bronchopneumonia it is frequently difficult to determine the causative organism because of the multiplicity of bacteria but infection is usually endogenous and most frequently caused by *Streptococcus pneumoniae*, *Staphylococcus aureus* and *Haemophilus influenzae*. Coliform organisms are also commonly involved. The course of the disease is unpredictable and the response to treatment is frequently capricious, unlike lobar pneumonia. In the latter young adults are often affected whereas in bronchopneumonia it is the young and old who succumb. Staphylococcal bronchopneumonia frequently follows influenza and bronchitis in the elderly and infirm and is a common cause of death

In children bronchopneumonia may follow whooping cough or a viral infection of the upper respiratory tract such as measles.

Laboratory diagnosis. A properly taken sample of sputum must be sent to the laboratory. Blood culture may also be useful in the diagnosis of lobar pneumonia.

Prophylaxis. This has been attempted by the use of vaccines containing prevalent pneumococcal types and a high degree of protection can be obtained by these. It is not a practicable proposition on a large scale but is useful for people at special risk.

Treatment. Antibiotic treatment will depend on sensitivity tests but penicillins are commonly used with a high measure of success.

Primary atypical pneumonia

Sometimes known as 'virus pneumonia' this is most commonly due to a bacterium-like organism *Mycoplasma pneumoniae*, although *Chlamydia* and *Coxiella* may also be associated with this type of infection. Infection is endemic in the community though epidemics can occur. *Mycoplasma pneumoniae* is cultured on enriched media and forms tiny colonies that may produce beta-haemolysis.

Diagnosis is by the complement-fixation test and this test should also be used to detect antibodies to *Chlamydia psittaci* and *Coxiella burneti*, the causative agents of psittacosis and Q fever respectively.

Mycoplasma pneumoniae is sensitive to erythromycin and tetracyclines.

Legionnaires' disease

Bacterial aetiology. *Legionella pneumophila*. A Gram-negative, non-acid-fast bacillus.

Pathogenesis and epidemiology. An explosive outbreak of severe pneumonia occurred in delegates attending an American Legion Convention in Philadelphia in 1976. Twenty nine of 182 cases were fatal. A retrospectively-diagnosed outbreak also occurred in Benidorm in 1973 and Pontiac in 1968 and many sporadic cases have been diagnosed all over the world since.

The mode of spread of this infection is airborne but not person to person. It is associated with cooling towers of air conditioning systems and with complex modern plumbing systems. The organisms exist in soil and ponds and when they reach the air cooling systems they are concentrated there and dispersed in aerosols. There is some evidence that the organisms may live in symbiosis with other bacteria and plants and they have been shown to be associated with the flowering of blue-green algae. In the Philadelphia outbreak many of the staff in the hotels where the delegates stayed had raised antibody titres to the organisms, suggesting that exposure may have been intermittent over several years and that asymptomatic infection is common. There is now increasing recognition of non-pulmonary disease such as intestinal and hepatic disorders and encephalopathy.

Laboratory diagnosis. The organism produces a characteristic disease in guinea pigs and death pattern in chick embryos after yolk-sac inoculation. Growth requirements are exacting; it fails to grow on ordinary bacteriological media but does so on special Mueller–Hinton medium. Immunofluorescent techniques can be used for diagnosis but may give false-positive results. Serology is the main diagnostic tool but by its nature it is restrospective.

Treatment. Legionnaire's disease should be treated with erythromycin with or without rifampicin. As the diagnosis is frequently delayed 'blind' therapy is often required.

Respiratory tuberculosis

Bacterial aetiology. Mycobacterium tuberculosis is the causative agent; *Mycobacterium bovis* no longer causes disease in the U.K.

(2) involvement of the regional mediastinal glands draining the primary focus.

In the majority of cases infection clears up spontaneously causing no symptoms but in some cases a more generalised infection may be produced either by direct spread causing tuberculous broncho-pneumonia, or by the haematogenous route causing miliary tuberculosis, affecting many sites.

Primary infection may occur via the intestinal tract if infected milk is drunk.

The mortality from tuberculosis has fallen dramatically since the middle of the last century (Fig. 16.5). Notification rates are also considerably lower, particularly in young children and young adults, formerly two of the most susceptible groups. Figs 16.6 and 16.7 show the pattern of tuberculosis in Scotland, 1972-80. At the present time tuberculosis is increasingly seen as an infection of the elderly.

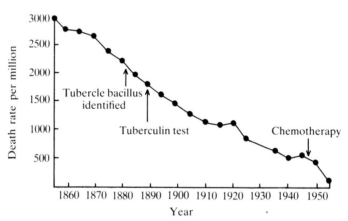

FIG. 16.5. Mean annual death rate for tuberculosis in England and Wales, 1860–1960.

Pathogenesis and epidemiology. The pathogenicity of tubercle bacilli depends on their ability to resist enzyme destruction in the macrophages. Intracellular growth occurs, the macrophages die and the bacilli either proceed to multiply extracellularly or, after ingestion by other macrophages, again intracellulary. Patients who recover naturally possess cell-mediated immunity and on re-exposure they have macrophages that have an enhanced ability to kill the organisms.

The most common form of primary infection is the production of the primary complex, comprising:

(1) a focus (Ghon) of infection in the subpleural area, probably at the site of implantation of the infecting bacilli.

Certain races seem to have a predisposition to tuberculosis.

Laboratory diagnosis. Tubercle bacilli are not commensal organisms and to isolate them from sputum is pathognomonic of the presence of tuberculous disease. Also, because saprophytic mycobacteria are rarely found in the respiratory tract the finding of even one acid-fast bacillus on a sputum smear stained by the Ziehl–Neelsen method is substantial evidence of pulmonary tuberculosis. Auramine staining is a more sensitive stain and is now much used. Such a provisional diagnosis is of immense importance as it allows chemotherapy to be started instantly without having to wait several weeks

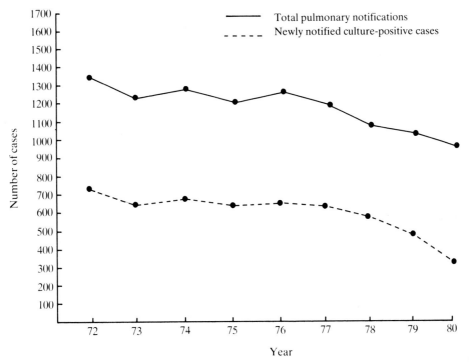

FIG. 16.6. Pulmonary tuberculosis in Scotland, 1972–80.

for the result of culture.

Sputum should be cultured on egg-containing media such as Löwenstein-Jensen or pyruvate medium, in screw-cap containers to preserve moisture over the long incubation period of six weeks.

Prophylaxis. This includes social measures such as better nutrition. The use of selective radiography as well as segregation and chemotherapy of known cases is important. The tuberculin test and administration of vaccine when required have also played a major role in the decrease in incidence of pulmonary tuberculosis.

The tuberculin test. The prevalence of tuberculosis can be measured by the tuberculin test which when positive indicates that the person has at some time been infected by *Mycobacterium tuberculosis*, without necessarily having symptoms and signs of the disease. Tuberculin testing checks for a delayed hypersensitivity reaction which indicates a degree of resistance to tuberculosis. Old tuberculin (OT), the

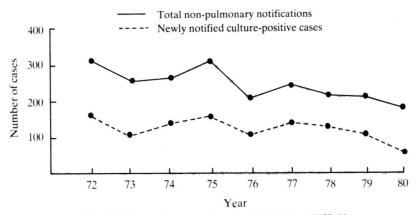

FIG. 16.7. Non-pulmonary tuberculosis in Scotland, 1972–80.

specific tuberculoprotein, or a purified protein derivative (PPD), is introduced into the skin of the forearm by intradermal injection (Mantoux test), or by multiple puncture (Heaf and Tine tests).

Whereas a positive result indicates that the person has had previous contact with infection or has had BCG vaccine and has therefore a degree of protection to tuberculosis, it can also mean that the person is currently suffering from the disease. A negative result usually excludes the disease although false negative results can be obtained in acute forms of the disease such as tuberculous meningitis or in the early stages of tuberculosis.

Vaccine. BCG (Bacille Calmette-Guérin) is a bovine strain of *Mycobacterium tuberculosis* attenuated by repeated growth on a bile-potato medium. The vaccine is given intradermally and current practice in the U.K. is that it should be offered to tuberculin-negative individuals who are at special risk, and also to tuberculin-negative schoolchildren between 10 and 13 years of age. The tuberculin test should always first be performed because of the risk of severe local reactions if BCG is given to a tuberculin-positive person. Complications of vaccinations are rare. Vaccine failures have been reported from time-to-time in the East.

Treatment. Isoniazid, para-amino salicylic acid, ethambutol, cycloserine, rifampicin, ethionamide and pyrazinamide can all be used. Frequently combinations of drugs are given. Because treatment has to be continued for many months repeated sputum cultures must be taken to ensure that they remain negative, as there is a tendency for drug resistance to occur.

Lung abscess

Bacterial aetiology. *Staphylococcus aureus*, *Streptococcus pyogenes*, *Streptococcus pneumoniae*, various Gram-negative bacilli and anaerobic organisms such as *Bacteroides* spp, *Fusobacterium* spp and anaerobic cocci may be involved.

Pathogenesis and epidemiology. A lung abscess is usually secondary to some pre-existing condition such as pneumonia, the presence of foreign bodies, trauma or tumours. The most common forms are those associated with pneumonia, although they are rarer nowadays because of more effective treatment of the primary cause.

Laboratory diagnosis. Sputum should be examined

and pus should be processed if available but it is also most important to diagnose the primary cause.

Treatment. Surgical treatment and drainage may be required and antibiotic therapy depends on the results of antibiograms.

Empyema

This is an abscess characterised by pus in the pleural space. An empyema is never primary and may be caused by:

(1) extension of lobar pneumonia, bronchopneumonia, tuberculosis or lung abscess.

(2) bacterial spread from the chest wall following thoracic surgery or trauma.

(3) spread of infection from below the diaphragm, as in hepatic or subphrenic abscess.

Pneumococci, staphylococci and *Haemophilus* organisms may be involved in spread from the lung; staphylococci and Gram-negative organisms from the chest wall; and coliform organisms and anaerobic cocci from under the diaphragm.

Pus must be aspirated and examined.

Psittacosis

Psittacosis, caused by chlamydiae, is a disease transmitted from birds to man. *Chlamydia psittaci* is common in birds and most infections are caused by parrots and budgerigars, by inhalation of infected material. The disease takes the form of primary atypical pneumonia.

Diagnosis. Complement fixation tests are the main methods of diagnosis.

Treatment. Tetracyclines or erythromycin may be used.

Q fever

Q ('query') fever is caused by a rickettsial organism *Coxiella burneti*. Animals, particularly sheep and cattle, are the reservoirs of the organisms and man is infected by inhalation of contaminated dust, by handling infected animals or by drinking unpasteurised milk from infected cattle.

Q fever is a generalised infection. Many people have a primary atypical pneumonia and rarely infective endocarditis may be caused.

Diagnosis, Complement fixation tests and guinea-pig inoculation are used.

Treatment. Chloramphenicol and tetracyclines are effective.

Respiratory Infection and Dentists

Respiratory tract infections are of particular concern to dentists as many of their patients will present for treatment while incubating, suffering from, or recovering from one. Transmission of infection is usually by the airborne route or by direct or indirect contact. Most infections will be produced by viruses which although generally not serious can cause considerable discomfort and often financial loss to the practitioner. Bacterial infections such as tuberculosis, diphtheria and whooping cough represent a serious health hazard to the dentist, the staff and fellow patients and no person suffering from one should be given dental treatment in general practice. Infections are not only spread from patient to dentist therefore any dentist with a severe respiratory tract infection should stay off work.

Risks of infection are enhanced by the use of aerosol-producing equipment such as air rotors, air and water syringes and ultrasonic scalers.

Dental surgery staff should be immunised against tuberculosis and diphtheria and should take common-sense precautions such as wearing masks, and, where necessary, gloves.

General anaesthesia should not be given to patients with respiratory infections because these give rise to obstruction, increased secretions and reduced respiratory efficiency.

FURTHER READING

Dubos R.J. & Hirsch J.G. (1965) *Bacterial and Mycotic Infections of Man*, 4th Edition. London, Pitman.

Duguid J.P., Marmion B.P. & Swain R.H.A. (1978) *Mackie and McCartney, Medical Microbiology*. 13th Edition. Edinburgh, Churchill Livingstone.

Fenner F. & White D.O. (1976) *Medical Virology*, 2nd Edition. London, Academic Press.

Horne N.W. (1971) Epidemiology and control of tuberculosis. *British Journal of Hospital Medicine*, **5**, 732–47.

Ross P.W. (1973) Problems in the diagnosis and treatment of the sore throat syndrome. *Pediatrics Digest*, **15**, 37–44.

Timbury M.C. (1978) *Notes on Medical Virology*, 6th Edition, Edinburgh, Churchill Livingstone.

Wannamaker L.W. (1972) Perplexity and precision in the diagnosis of streptococcal pharyngitis. *American Journal of Diseases of Children*, **124**, 352–8.

CHAPTER 17

Infections of the Cardiovascular System

Defences against infection

Portals of entry to the bloodstream are the skin, mucosae, the genitourinary, respiratory and intestinal tracts.

The body's normal defence mechanisms may be upset by several factors:

(1) disturbance of the normal protective flora of the various areas of the body by the administration of broad-spectrum antibiotics,

(2) variations in the immune state of the host due top steroid therapy immunosuppression, immune deficiency diseases, metabolic diseases, irradiation, blood dyscrasias and malignancies.

Potential pathogens (Fig. 17.1).

Bacteraemia and septicaemia

Bacteraemia is simply the presence of bacteria in the blood and is a common occurrence. It can be produced merely by brushing teeth, or chewing, or by diagnostic procedures such as sigmoidoscopy and urinary tract catheterisation. It is generally a transient phenomenon as the bacteria are not actively multiplying and are quickly removed by the action of the host defences. Conversely, when large numbers of bacteria enter the bloodstream and actively multiply a septicaemia is produced. This is quite different from a simple bacteraemia because the patient is clinically ill, often with focal infection in some organ, and the infection will progress unless controlled by antimicrobial drugs, with or without surgical intervention.

Organisms isolated from blood

The most common isolates of clinical significance are *Staphylococcus aureus* and Gram-negative bacilli, including *Escherichia coli, Proteus, Pseudomonas, Klebsiella, Salmonella, Haemophilus, Bacteroides* and *Brucella. Streptococci,* particularly the viridans streptococci, *Streptococcus pneumoniae* and *Streptococcus faecalis* are also common isolates. Neisseriae, clostridia, anaerobic cocci, *Staphylococcus albus* and *Candida albicans* are less commonly found.

Predisposing factors

Peripheral sources include injury to the skin, for example surgical wounds, dental extractions, intravenous tubes, haemodialysis, injection sites, burns and graft infections.

Central sources include therapeutic trauma such as sigmoidoscopy or even enemas, jejunal biopsy, catheterisation of the bladder, dilatation of the urethra, dental extraction, cardiac catheterisation and pacemaker wires. Collections of pus under pressure and infected tumours are also potential sources. In the patient receiving immunosuppressive drugs, cytoxic drugs or corticosteroids, 'the compromised host', the immune mechanisms are less able to cope with invading organisms and organisms of lesser pathogenicity can produce septicaemia.

Infective endocarditis

Microbial aetiology. Oral streptococci, especially *Streptococcus sanguis* and *mitior* and *Streptococcus*

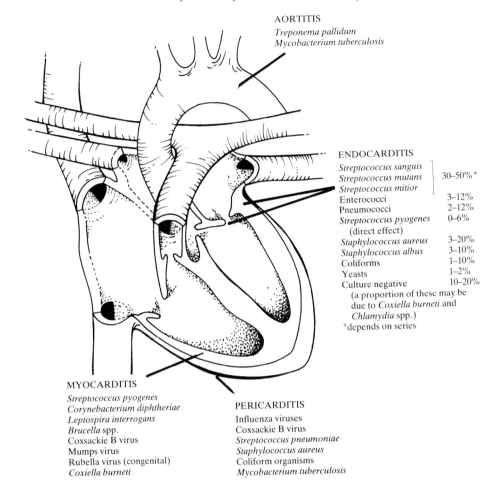

AORTITIS
Treponema pallidum
Mycobacterium tuberculosis

ENDOCARDITIS

Streptococcus sanguis	
Streptococcus mutans	30–50%*
Streptococcus mitior	
Enterococci	3–12%
Pneumococci	2–12%
Streptococcus pyogenes	0–6%
(direct effect)	
Staphylococcus aureus	3–20%
Staphylococcus albus	3–10%
Coliforms	1–10%
Yeasts	1–2%
Culture negative	10–20%

(a proportion of these may be
due to *Coxiella burneti* and
Chlamydia spp.)
*depends on series

MYOCARDITIS
Streptococcus pyogenes
Corynebacterium diphtheriae
Leptospira interrogans
Brucella spp.
Coxsackie B virus
Mumps virus
Rubella virus (congenital)
Coxiella burneti

PERICARDITIS
Influenza viruses
Coxsackie B virus
Streptococcus pneumoniae
Staphylococcus aureus
Coliform organisms
Mycobacterium tuberculosis

FIG. 17.1 Pathogens of the heart and great vessels.

faecalis are most frequently involved. Other less common streptococci are *Streptococcus mutans*, *milleri* and *salivarius*. Other bacteria associated with infective endocarditis include staphylococci, *Haemophilus* spp, anaerobic cocci, *Bacteroides* spp and Gram-negative rods such as *Escherichia coli*, *Klebsiella*, *Pseudomonas* and *Proteus* spp. The pyogenic cocci are generally involved in the more acute forms.

Non-bacterial causes are less common and such organisms are *Coxiella burneti*, *Chlamydia psittaci*, *Candida* and other fungi. The latter are commonly isolated after open-heart surgery.

Viruses are not thought to be causes of infective endocarditis.

Pathogenesis and epidemiology. Acute and subacute forms can occur and because at times the line of demarcation between the two is difficult to draw, it is advisable to call the condition 'infective endocarditis' rather than the hitherto commonly used terms of 'acute' and 'subacute' endocarditis.

Infective endocarditis has been known to occur in patients with apparently normal valves but in general the condition occurs in those with some pathology of the endocardium, such as damage to the valve from pre-existing rheumatic fever, valve prostheses, septal defects, atheroma of the valve and congenital valve deformities. Even minor degenerative changes in the aortic and mitral valves carry a risk for the elderly. Generally only one organism is involved but mixed

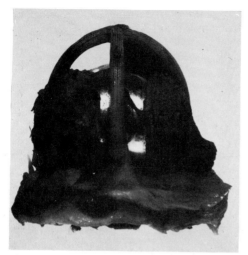

FIG. 17.2 This Starr-Edwards valve was removed at autopsy. It shows the fabric-covered cruciform cage which retains the light interior ball. Note the pillars of laminated thrombus (vegetations) occupying regions between the radii and circumference of the cage.

infections can occur in the compromised host and in 'mainline' drug addicts. Mixed infections add considerably to the problems of diagnosis and treatment.

A sterile platelet-fibrin thrombus develops on a valve and organisms then become implanted in the thrombus as the result of bacteraemia. Organisms grow and produce fragile vegetations from which emboli are constantly shed. Vegetations comprise fibrin, platelets and organisms. The avascularity of the thrombi reduces the effectiveness of anti-microbial therapy. In fatal cases death is commonly due to congestive cardiac failure or to valve perforation. Fig 17.2 shows an artificial valve removed at autopsy and Fig. 17.3 shows the artificial ball case with thrombus.

Endocarditis can occur at any age, although in recent times there has been a marked change in the age group affected; hitherto those up to and around 30 years of age comprised those most commonly afflicted but nowadays inefective endocarditis is more a disease of the elderly in whom enterococci are becoming increasingly the infecting agents.

Accurate figures for the incidence of the disease are unknown because it does not have to be notified. The mortality rate is high, between 20 and 30 per cent, and this is partly accounted for by late diagnosis and poor management. It is believed that between 30-50 per cent of cases have a history of receiving dental treatment, some as long as three months before the attack. The definition of 'treatment' is often vague and the precise relationship between any particular form of dental treatment and the onset of endocarditis remains unsolved. The link with dental extractions may be quite clear, however, and the oral origin of most bacteria isolated from the blood of

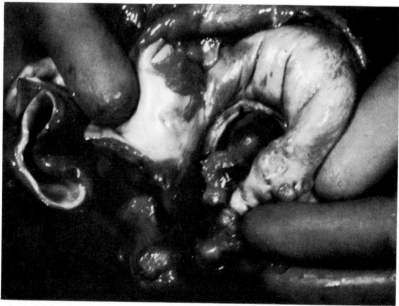

FIG. 17.3. This shows the aorta opened from above. The periphery of the prosthetic valve is clearly seen, occupying the position of removed aortic cusps. The cruciform nature of the ball cage is largely obscured by masses of thrombus (vegetations). Courtesy of Dr. S. Fletcher.

patients with infective endocarditis greatly implicates dental treatment of poor oral health in the aetiology of this condition. The majority of the remainder give a history of some genitourinary or gastrointestinal intervention.

Laboratory examination. This is one of the many infections where close collaboration between ward and laboratory is vital in diagnosis and in the control of antimicrobial chemotherapy. Blood culture is the main diagnostic procedure and should be done without delay in any patient who has an unexplained pyrexia and who is known to have some cardiac lesion.

Blood culture. Bacteria can be isolated from first cultures in more than 80 per cent of patients with infective endocarditis and bacteraemia is often more persistent than intermittent. Many media can be used for culture of blood, such as cooked meat broth, brain heart infusion and thiol broth. It is important to subculture on to solid media and incubate both aerobically and anaerobically.

If blood cultures remain negative and there is strong clinical evidence of endocarditis serological tests should be done for antibodies against *Chlamydia, Coxiella burneti*, and fungi. If valve replacement is required the diseased valve should be sent for culture.

Culture-negative endocarditis. About 20 per cent of blood cultures remain negative.

Several reasons are suggested for this:

(1) chemotherapy has been started.

(2) bacteraemia is intermittent and an inadequate number of specimens has been taken.

(3) organisms may be fastidious or slow growers like *Bacteroides* spp.

(4) rickettsiae, *Coxiella* or chlamydiae may be involved; serological tests will clarify.

(5) L-forms of the organisms may be present.

(6) bacteria may be sequestered in the vegetations.

Points to note in taking blood for culture. Take blood before any chemotherapy, preferably 3–4 paired cultures per day at intervals. Paired cultures are useful in checking for contaminants. Blood can be taken at any time. The site of venepuncture must be adequately cleansed. Use a bottle containing penicillinase if the patient is on penicillin or ampicillin. Most laboratories have an incubator available for blood cultures taken outwith laboratory hours. When blood is taken the needle should be changed before inoculating the broth medium; this will minimise the risk of contamination.

Treatment. In severe cases treatment must start after one blood culture has been taken; the disease is far too serious to wait for laboratory diagnosis. A combination of bactericidal drugs should be used; bacteriostatic drugs will not kill organisms that are embedded in vegetations. Combinations of a penicillin (benzyl penicillin, amoxycillin or ampicillin) and an aminoglycoside (gentamicin or streptomycin) are widely used and are very effective.

Laboratory control of treatment is essential. Measurement of the minimum inhibitory concentration (MIC) of the antibiotic combination should be made. Peak and trough levels of serum antibiotic must be measured to ensure that these levels are adequate to allow penetration of the vegetations and kill the organisms. Treatment must last for at least six weeks. If relatively toxic antibiotics such as gentamicin are used serum levels must be monitored daily and adjustments to the dose may have to be made.

In *Coxiella burneti* infection surgical excision of the valve is usually required with long-term treatment with tetracyclines or clindamycin.

Operation for valve insertion should be carried out after a normal course of treatment which should be continued for another two weeks. In some cases emergency valve replacement has been carried out successfully before the infective episode is over. Careful control of antibiotic therapy is required but results are encouraging. It is important that patients undergoing valve replacement surgery, whether as an emergency or a planned procedure, have good dental health and are capable of maintaining this. These patients require long-term follow-up care and this and the operation itself are costly. It is obviously unwise for a patient with a replaced valve to suffer episodes of bacteraemia from chronic periodontal disease or dental abscesses. There is some evidence for such patients being more at risk of developing more severe infective endocarditis than those with congenital abnormalities or a history of rheumatic fever who have not had valve surgery. The American Heart Association includes such patients in a special 'at risk' category warranting a separate prophylatic antibiotic protocol. Patients with poor dentition and those unwilling to maintain good health prior to valve surgery should probably have all remaining teeth extracted. This is not a complete guarantee of avoiding endocarditis as some patients develop infective endocarditis with an organism of non-oral origin or from an ulcer in the oral mucosa.

Prophylaxis of infective endocarditis

Prophylaxis and dentistry. The American Heart Association periodically produces authoritative statements on recommended prophylactic antibiotic regimens for patients at risk of developing infective endocarditis. This Association stresses:

(1) the importance of parenteral antibiotics especially for patients in high-risk groups such as those with prosthetic valves,

(2) close co-operation between physicians and dentists in the management of these patients,

(3) the need for these patients to maintain 'the highest level of oral health' even in edentulous patients who wear dentures.

There is considerable evidence to show that all of these recommendations are ignored to some degree. The 1977 recommendations for antibiotic prophylaxis for dental surgery are given in Table 17.1. Regimen A is for general prophylaxis. Regimen B is required for all patients with prosthetic heart valves; antibiotic prophylaxis is recommended before any procedure that is likely to result in gingival bleeding, except for the natural shedding of deciduous teeth or the adjustment of orthodontic appliances.

The important points to note are that antibiotics are given only 30 minutes to one hour before surgery and are continued for a maximum of only two days after surgery. This is intended to prevent the selection of resistant strains from which bacteraemia may arise. Bactericidal antibiotics should be used; bacteriostatic agents such as tetracycline are inappropriate drugs.

Because it is impossible to obtain universal adoption of the recommendation of the American Heart Association outlined in Table 17.1 modifications of this have been proposed. Many dentists find that cooperation with cardiologists is poor and dentists often lack training and experience in administering parenteral antibiotics. Recently amoxycillin, a modification of ampicillin, has been recommended as a prophylatic antibiotic that can be administered as a single 3g oral dose (Table 17.2).

TABLE 17.1. The American Heart Association recommended prophylactic antibiotic regimens for dentists.

REGIMEN A

Parenteral and oral penicillin

Adults: 1 000 000 U penicillin G mixed with } intramuscularly ½ – 1 h
600 000 U procaine penicillin } prior to procedure
plus 500 mg phenoxymethyl penicillin (Pen V) : 4 × daily for 2 days

Children: 30 000 U/kg penicillin G mixed } intramuscularly as for adults
with 600 000 U procaine penicillin }

plus 250 mg phenoxymethyl penicillin (Pen V) : 4× daily for 2 days.

Patients allergic to penicillin

Adults: 1 g erythromycin — orally 1½–2 h prior to procedure
plus 500 mg erythromycin — orally 4 ×daily for 2 days
Children: 20 mg/kg erythromycin — orally } timing as for adults
plus 10 mg/kg erythromycin — orally }

REGIMEN B : PATIENTS WITH PROSTHETIC VALVES

Penicillin and streptomycin

Adults: 1 000 000 U penicillin G mixed with }
600 000 U procaine penicillin } all intramuscularly ½–1 h prior to procedure
plus 1 g streptomycin }
plus 500 mg phenoxymethyl penicillin : 4 × daily for 2 days
Children: 30 000 U/kg penicillin G mixed with } timing as for adults
600 000 U procaine penicillin }
plus 250 mg phenoxymethyl penicillin, timing as for adults

For patients allergic to penicillin

Adults: 1 g vancomycin — intravenously by slow infusion lasting ½–1 h and given prior to procedure
plus 500 mg erythromycin orally — 4 × daily for 2 days
Children: 20 mg/kg vancomycin intravenously } timing of doses as for adults
plus 10 mg/kg erythromycin orally }

N.B. Intravenous vancomycin is recommended by the American Heart Association as an alternative for patients allergic to penicillin but this is not widely accepted.

TABLE 17.2. Other suitable prophylactic regimens for dental procedures in susceptible patients.

Amoxycillin in high dose
   Adults: 3g orally 1 h prior to procedure followed by
                    3g 8 h after procedure
   Children (up to 12 years):   1.5 g orally 1 h prior to procedure followed by
                                            1.5 g 8 h after procedure

Erythromycin (for patients allergic to penicillin)
Oral only — see regimen A Table 17.1
   Adults (parenteral):   300 mg by slow intravenous injection
                                   plus 500 mg orally 4 × daily for 2 days
   Child (parenteral):   150 mg by slow intravenous injection
                                   plus 250 mg orally 4 × daily for 2 days

Penicillin and gentamicin
   1 000 000 U penicillin G mixed with 600 000 U procaine penicillin, all intramuscularly

   plus 80 mg gentamicin
   plus 500 mg phenoxymethyl penicillin   :   4 × daily for 2 days

Vancomycin and gentamicin
   1 g vancomycin by slow intravenous injection ½ – 1 h prior to procedure
   80 mg gentamicin intramuscularly 30 min prior to procedure and 80 mg 8 h after procedure.

However, it may be wise to give a second 3g dose after 6–8 hours. The obvious appeal of such a simple regimen may lead to its being used more widely than the parenteral regimens. It has not yet, however, been fully tested in animal models of endocarditis. Clinical trials of prophylactic regimens for endocarditis are almost impossible to conduct because of the uncertainty of predicting which patient will develop endocarditis.

Patients allergic to penicillins have usually been given erythromycin in some form. While this is reasonable the high oral doses (2–3g) are likely to cause considerable gastrointestinal discomfort; intramuscular injection is painful and intravenous injection is most unlikely to be practised by a dentist. The ideal regimen is far from clear but the parenteral and oral penicillin combination of regimen A (Table 17.1) with oral erythromycin as an alternative seems useful and practical. Patients receiving a general anaesthetic should get parenteral penicillin preoperatively or erythromycin if allergic to penicillin. Oral penicillin or erythromycin can be given postoperatively. A protocol to help choose an appropriate regimen is given in Table 17.3.

TABLE 17.3. Suggested protocol for choosing appropriate regimen

		Table
(i) For routine use	Parenteral and oral penicillin	17.1
	Or amoxycillin high dose	17.2
For patients allergic to penicillin	Parenteral or oral erythromycin	17.1
(ii) For patients with prosthetic valves	Parenteral penicillin and gentamicin plus oral penicillin	17.2
For patients allergic to penicillin	*Parenteral vancomycin and gentamicin	17.2
(iii) For patients about to undergo general anaesthesia	Parenteral and oral penicillin	17.1
For patients allergic to penicillin	Parenteral and oral erythromycin	17.2
(iv) For patients with prosthetic valves about to undergo general anaesthesia	Parenteral penicillin and gentamicin plus oral penicillin	17.2
For patients allergic to penicillin	Parenteral vancomycin plus gentamicin	17.2

* These patients should preferably be admitted to hospital day-bed units. Injection or infusion of vancomycin should not be carried out in a general dental practice even by a medical practitioner.

Prophylaxis and other procedures. Penicillin with streptomycin or gentamicin, or ampicillin and gentamicin, are suitable combinations for those undergoing urinary or intestinal tract manipulations because of their effect against *Streptococcus faecalis*.

In those about to undergo cardiac surgery a combination of benzyl penicillin or flucloxacillin and an aminoglycoside such as gentamicin will be effective against most relevant pathogenic bacteria.

Myocarditis

Many causes of this disease are not of microbial origin but diphtheria, trypanosomiasis, toxoplasmosis, leptospirosis and virus infections such as influenza and coxsackie B can produce it.

Pericarditis

Viruses, such as influenza and coxsackie B, are the most common causes. Bacteria such as staphylococci, pneumococci and *Mycobacterium tuberculosis* may cause the disease either as a complication of septicaemia or by direct extension from an intrathoracic infection, but only very rarely.

Rheumatic fever (RF)

This is not in itself an infectious disease. It is caused by an adverse immune response to *Streptococcus pyogenes*, the nature of which is still unclear. The generally-accepted theory of its production is that antibodies to streptococcal antigens cross react with myocardial antigens. Immune complexes and cell-mediated reactions may also be involved and there may well be a genetic component. Rheumatic fever is a pancarditis but the residual damage is to the heart valves. It is these damaged valves that are very susceptible to infective endocarditis. As well as the above example there is other evidence of the connection between *Streptococcus pyogenes* and RF, namely clinical, epidemological, serological and chemoprophylactic.

Clinical. RF occurs a few weeks after an attack of scarlet fever and patients often admit having had a sore throat several weeks before the onset of RF.

Epidemiological. RF rates increase when the streptococcal carriage rate increases and in the U.K. the age group which has the highest incidence of RF (seven to nine years) is also that which has the highest incidence of streptococcal sore throat.

Serological. RF does not occur in the absence of immunological evidence of streptococcal infection. The first antibody to be measured was anti-streptolysin O (ASO); titres become detectable in the second week after the onset of infection, are maximal by the sixth week and thereafter decrease. Other titres such as antihyaluroidase (AH), antistreptokinase (ASK), antideoxyribonuclease B (Anti DNAse B) and antinicotinamide adenine dinucleotisdase (Anti-NADase) can be measured, but most laboratories perform only the ASO and sometimes the anti DNAse B tests. Fig. 17.4 shows the percentage of patients with raised antibodies according to the number of serological tests performed.

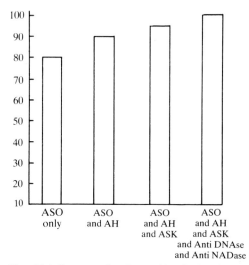

FIG. 17.4. Per cent of patients with raised antibody titre in early stages of rheumatic fever.

Chemoprophylaxis. RF in the U.K. is very much on the decline and the incidence of primary attacks is considerably less than 0.5 per cent. To prevent these is virtually impossible. Penicillin treatment of streptococcal sore throat has been said to be of value in prevention but there is a great deal of evidence to show that this plays little part. For example, the incidence of RF in the U.K. had greatly decreased before the advent of antibiotics and also only a fraction of the population with streptoccal infection is treated with antibiotics since infection may be subclinical. Prevention of second or subsequent attacks of RF is quite a different matter because the person who has had a primary attack of RF is prone to further attacks and undoubtedly daily prophylaxis using oral penicillin, or erythromycin in cases of hypersensitivity to penicillin, has proved of great benefit to these children.

It must be remembered that although the incidence of RF has decreased markedly in the West it is still a major problem in developing countries.

FURTHER READING

American Heart Association Committee Report (1977) Prevention of bacterial endocarditis. *Circulation* **56**, 139A–43A.

Cawson R. (1982) *The Nature and Prevention of Bacterial Endocarditis.* Medicine Publishing Foundation Symposium Series 3. Oxford. Medicine Publishing Foundation.

Garrod L.P., Lambert H.P. & O'Grady F. (1981) *Antibiotic and Chemotherapy,* 5th Edition. Edinburgh, Churchill Livingstone.

Hayward G.W. (1973) Infective endocarditis: a changing disease. *British Medical Journal* **2,** 706–9: 764–6.

Holbrook W.P., Willey R.F. & Shaw T.R.D. (1981) Dental health in patients susceptible to infective endocarditis. *British Medical Journal,* **283,** 371–2.

Holbrook W.P., Willey R.F. & Shaw T.R.D. (1983) Prophylaxis of infective endocarditis: Problems in practice. *British Dental Journal,* **154,** 36–9.

Oakley C.M. (1980) Infective endocarditis. *British Journal of Hospital Medicine,* **24,** 232–43.

Wannamaker L.W. & Matsen J.M. (1972) *Streptococci and Streptococcal Diseases.* London. Academic Press.

Working Party of the British Society for Antimicrobial Chemotherapy. (1982). The antibiotic prophylaxis of infective endocarditis. *Lancet* **ii,** 1323–6.

CHAPTER 18

Infections of the Central Nervous System and Locomotor System

CENTRAL NERVOUS SYSTEM (CNS)

Defences against infection

The cerebrospinal fluid (CSF) does not contain any effective antibacterial substances and since there are no other local defences infection rapidly becomes generalised when a pyogenic organism gains access to the subarachnoid space and the cerebrospinal fluid, by direct extension or via the blood.

Potential pathogens (Fig. 18.1).

Acute pyogenic meningitis (also called acute bacterial or acute purulent meningitis).

Bacterial aetiology. Table 18.1 shows the causes of acute bacterial meningitis in England, Wales and Ireland from 1976–80.

Pathogenesis and epidemiology

(1) *Neonatal meningitis.* Although in former years this was commonly caused by *Streptococcus pyogenes* and *Staphylococcus aureus,* coliform bacilli have been important causes in the last two decades. In recent years, group B streprococci have been responsible for many cases of neonatal meningitis and at present they rival the coliform organisms in being the most common causative agents. Coliform meningitis often results from congenital deformities such as spina bifida, and the sources of the organisms can be the genitourinary tract, lungs or umbilicus. Two forms of group B streptococcal meningitis are recognised; the early-onset form that occurs within 36 hours of birth and in which infection is contracted from the cervicovaginal canal of the mother, and the late-onset form that does not usually occur until 10 days or more after birth and which is likely to be nosocomial in origin.

(2) *Haemophilus meningitis.* Although adult cases have been described this mostly occurs in young children between the ages of three months and five years. Protection before three months is provided by maternal antibody and after five years by acquired immunity. Infection is spread by the bloodstream from some focus such as an upper respiratory tract infection. Capsulate organisms of Pittman's type b are most commonly responsible for these infections. Penicillinase-producing strains are now presenting treatment problems.

(3) *Meningococcal meningitis.* Meningococci enter the body via the nasopharynx where they may either produce a localised inflammatory reaction or remain quiescent. There are two main theories as to how they reach the meninges:

(a) that they spread by direct extension along the spaces between the sheath and the branches of the olfactory nerve that pierce the cribriform plate, and

(b) the more likely theory, that the organisms invade the bloodstream and either produce a transient bacteraemia or multiply in the blood and cause metastatic lesions elsewhere in the body, such as in the skin, adrenal glands, joints and meninges. Nine groups of meningococci (A–D; X, Y, Z, Z^1, W135) are recognised; group B is the most common in the U.K.

Infection is most readily spread in conditions of close household contact.

Prophylaxis of meningococcal meningitis. No antibiotic is totally effective in eliminating the carrier state but rifampicin or minocycline may be used.

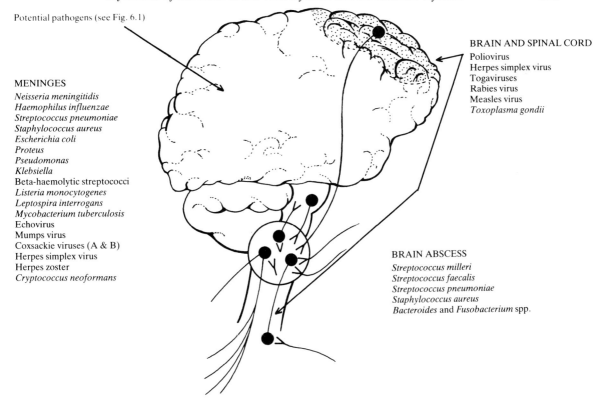

FIG. 18.1. Potential pathogens of the central nervous system.

Potential pathogens (see Fig. 6.1)

MENINGES

Neisseria meningitidis
Haemophilus influenzae
Streptococcus pneumoniae
Staphylococcus aureus
Escherichia coli
Proteus
Pseudomonas
Klebsiella
Beta-haemolytic streptococci
Listeria monocytogenes
Leptospira interrogans
Mycobacterium tuberculosis
Echovirus
Mumps virus
Coxsackie viruses (A & B)
Herpes simplex virus
Herpes zoster
Cryptococcus neoformans

BRAIN AND SPINAL CORD

Poliovirus
Herpes simplex virus
Togaviruses
Rabies virus
Measles virus
Toxoplasma gondii

BRAIN ABSCESS

Streptococcus milleri
Streptococcus faecalis
Streptococcus pneumoniae
Staphylococcus aureus
Bacteroides and *Fusobacterium* spp.

Vaccines produced from strains of groups A and C have proved efective in the U.S.A. and Brazil and group A vaccine has been used.

(4) *Pneumococcal meningitis.* This may be caused either by septicaemic spread secondary to conditions such as lobar pneumonia or otitis media, or by direct infection from the paranasal sinuses following injury to the skull. It carries a high mortality rate in elderly patients.

(5) *Meningitis due to other bacteria.* These include *Staphylococcus aureus* and *Streptococcus pyogenes.* They reach the meninges either via the bloodstream, by direct extension from the ear or paranasal sinuses, or directly from the exterior after trauma.

(6) *Tuberculous meningitis.* This occurs in a particularly severe form in young children between two and five years of age and is probably secondary to a tuberculous focus elsewhere in the body usually the

TABLE 18.1. The major causes of bacterial meningitis reported in England, Wales and Ireland in 1976–80.

Causative organism	Number of cases in the stated year			
	1976	1978	1979	1980
Neisseria meningitidis	571	401	461	412
Haemophilus spp.	320	282	337	443
Streptococcus pneumoniae	239	292	307	307
Escherichia coli and coliform organisms*	108	88	71	89
Staphylococci	64	88	80	69
Streptococci (excluding pneumococci)	51	81	86	95
Mycobacterium tuberculosis	23	31	18	25
Totals	1376	1263	1360	1440

* Other cases were caused by *Proteus, Klebsiella, Pseudomonas* spp. etc.

TABLE 18.2. The cerebrospinal fluid in meningitis.

	Normal	Acute pyogenic	Tuberculous	Aseptic
Appearance	Clear	Turbid	Clear or opalescent	Usually clear
Total protein	15–40 mg/100 ml	Greatly increased; 200–600 mg/100 ml	Increased	Normal
Sugar	50–70 mg/100 ml	Greatly reduced or absent	Reduced	Normal
Lactate	Normal	Raised	Considerably raised	Normal
Cell count	0–3 lymphocytes/cu mm	Greatly increased; polymorphs	Increased; mainly lymphocytes but some polymorphs	Increased; lymphocytes

lung. The bacilli reach the meninges via the bloodstream.

(7) *Listeria monocytogenes* and *Leptospira interrogans* are rare causes of meningitis.

Laboratory diagnosis of meningitis. Various changes occur in the cerebrospinal fluid depending on whether the aetiology is acute pyogenic, tuberculous or viral (Table 18.2).

Blood cultures are particularly useful in the diagnosis of bacterial meningitis and may be positive in approximately 50 per cent of cases. A five ml volume of cerebrospinal fluid is removed by lumbar puncture and a cell count made. The fluid is centrifuged and Gram films are made from the deposit (Ziehl-Neelsen if tuberculous meningitis is suspected). Microscopy may be sufficient to indicate the diagnosis and to allow chemotherapy to commence but cultures are also made on blood agar, chocolate agar and on New York City medium which is selective for neisseriae. They are incubated up to 24 hours in an atmosphere of 10 per cent carbon dioxide. Biochemical and/or serological tests confirm the identity of the organism. For tuberculous meningitis Löwenstein-Jensen slopes are set up and guinea pigs inoculated.

Treatment. Chemotherapy will depend on the nature of the organism and the antibiogram, but as this infection is a medical emergency two or even three antibiotics are often given initially; these include a penicillin and chloramphenicol.

Viral meningitis (aseptic meningitis).

Aetiology. Table 18.3 shows the main causes of viral meningitis and/or encephalitis reported in Great Britain in 1979.

TABLE 18.3. The major causes of viral meningitis and/or encephalitis reported in Great Britian in 1979. From Noah N.D. & Urquhart A.M. (1980). Virus meningitis and encephalitis in 1979. *Journal of Infection* 2, 379–83.

Virus	Number of cases
Echovirus	386
Mumps virus	317
Coxsackie virus	154
Herpes simplex virus	125
Adenovirus	43
Measles virus	42
Influenza virus	38
Varicella-zoster virus	33

Pathogenesis and epidemiology. Viruses enter the body principally by the respiratory or gastrointestinal tracts. Spread to the central nervous system (CNS) may be by migration within nerves by the olfactory route or in most cases by the blood. Viruses gain entry to the CNS by way of the capillary endothelial cells, by infected leucocytes or by the epithelial cells of the choroid plexus. Children and young adults are mostly affected. There is no specific treatment; antiviral agents are not prescribed and the condition generally resolves in two weeks.

Encephalitis

It is customary to separate infection of the meninges from encephalitis which is an infection of the brain substance but to a certain extent this is an artificial distinction because patients often have symptoms and signs that relate to both these areas.

Aetiology. Herpes simplex, mumps and arboviruses are most frequently involved in viral encephalitis.

Postinfectious encephalitis occurs after childhood illnesses such as measles, chickenpox and rubella. Postvaccinial encephalitis may be a sequel to immunisation with live viral vaccines such as vaccinia, yellow fever and measles, and inactivated vaccines such as pertussis.

Unlike viral meningitis viral encephalitis is a very serious disease with significant mortality and morbidity.

Blood can be collected for virus isolation and brain biopsy material can be examined in immuno-fluorescence techniques.

Treatment. Viral encephalitis is one of the rare indications for specific antiviral therapy (Chap. 11).

Poliomyelitis

Aetiology. Poliovirus, types 1–3.

Pathogenesis and epidemiology. Poliovirus, an enterovirus, enters the body via the mouth and multiplies in the lymphoid tissue of the pharynx and intestine. A viraemia then occurs and the viruses may then spread to the CNS producing neurological disease. In most case a febrile influenza-like illness is caused although an aseptic meningitis may occur in some people. Very few contract poliomyelitis, the paralytic disease. With the advent of poliovaccine cases are now rare in the developed countries, but the disease is prevalent in the Third World.

Cerebral abscess

The following bacteria may cause this condition: *Streptococcus milleri, Streptococcus faecalis/faecium, Streptococcus pneumoniae, Staphylococcus aureus, Bacteroides* spp. anaerobic cocci and coliforms. Infections are frequently mixed.

Pathogenesis and epidemiology. Abscess formation can occur via the bloodstream or as the result of direct extension into the brain. To a degree the types of bacteria are related to the source of the infection and the route of spread determines the site of the abscess. The sources of infection vary and include otitis media, sinusitis and metastatic spread from chest infection. Infection may also follow dental, abdominal or neurological surgery and may occur after head injuries. Temporal lobe or cerebellar hemisphere abscesses are associated with otitis media and mastoiditis and frontal lobe abscesses with infection of the ethmoidal, sphenoidal and frontal sinuses. Frontal lobe abscesses can also be a rare complication of acute and chronic dental infection.

Laboratory diagnosis. The most reliable measure is to obtain pus by aspiration or at operation. Stained smears of the untreated pus should be examined and aerobic and anaerobic culture of the pus undertaken.

Treatment. Where practicable excision of abscesses is mandatory and antibiotics must be given. The penicillin group and gentamicin are widely used, and metronidazole should always be considered because of the frequent associations of *Bacteroides fragilis* and other anaerobic bacteria with cerebral abscess. In addition metronidazole penetrates well into abscesses.

Tetanus

Bacterial aetiology. Clostridium tetani.

Pathogenesis and epidemiology. Tetanus is the result of contamination of a wound with *Clostridium tetani* spores, frequently from manured soil, contaminated dust or clothing. Germination of the spores in a wound depends on reduced oxygen tension which can occur in any devitalised tissue and which may also be produced if aerobes multiply concomitantly in the wound. *Clostridium tetani* remains localised in the wound but when the spores germinate a potent diffusible toxin is produced which is absorbed at the motor nerve endings and travels by way of the motor nerves to the anterior horn cells of the spinal cord. The nearer the wound is to the head (face, upper limbs) the more serious the disease. The exotoxin is a protein and has two components, tetanospasmin and tetanolysin.

Although tetanus is commonly associated with deep wounds it can nevertheless result from superficial abrasions, including scratches and rose-thorn pricks.

Laboratory diagnosis. Although diagnosis is essentially clinical Gram films should be made from the wound exudate and examined for 'drum-stick' bacilli. Special stains can reveal the characteristic terminal spore. The bacilli grow well on blood-containing media under strict anaerobic conditions. Biochemical tests can confirm their identity and animal inoculation can test for toxigenicity of the organism.

Prophylaxis

(1) *Prevention of germination of tetanus spores.* This includes prompt and thorough wound toilet and surgical debridement if required.

(2) *Provision of sufficient antitoxin to neutralise any*

tetanus toxin that may be produced. This can be done either by giving:

    (a) a booster dose of tetanus toxoid to those already actively immunised, or

    (b) anti-tetanus serum (ATS) (or human anti-tetanus globulin (ATG)) to those not actively immunised.

ATG should be used in preference to ATS because of the risk of hypersensitivity reactions in patients given horse antiserum. ATG is freely available in the U.K. but this situation may not apply in developing countries. Combined active-passive immunisation must be given to the non-immune person; this gives immediate passive protection by the ATG while active immunity is developing.

    (3) *Prevention of multiplication (and therefore toxin production) of the vegetative bacilli.* This can be achieved by giving prophylactic antibiotics (penicillin) (and can replace 2b), although the use of both procedures is recommended. In casualty departments penicillin is usually given not just to prevent tetanus but to prevent a pyogenic infection.

Treatment. As well as general measures such as the use of muscle relaxants, sedation and artificial ventilation, antitoxin can be given although this is of little use if the toxin has become fixed to the tissues. Those who recover from tetanus require a course of active immunisation because the disease does not produce immunity.

THE LOCOMOTOR SYSTEM

Defences against infection

In the joint these include the synovial membrane and its cells which are specialised macrophages with a highly phagocytic action. Synovial fluid contains a few mononuclear cells, some complement and lysozyme.

Potential pathogens (Fig. 18.2)

Acute septic arthritis

Bacterial aetiology. Bacteria commonly associated with this infection are *Staphylococcus aureus, Haemophilus influenzae,* Beta-haemolytic streptococci and neisseriae, together with rarer causes such as *Brucella* and *Salmonella* spp and non-sporing anaerobes such as *Bacteroides* spp.

Pathogenesis and epidemiology. Infection can occur by:

    (1) penetrating injury through joint capsule.

    (2) secondary direct spread from a nearby focus of infection such as osteomyelitis.

    (3) haematogenous spread to the capillary network in the synovial membrane and hence to the joint.

The knee joints are most frequently affected, then the hip and ankle.

Sources of septic arthritis are numerous and include sepsis of the skin, nasopharynx, sinuses, lung, peritoneum and genital tract. Acute septic arthritis occurs most commonly in children. In an infant under six months of age the most likely organisms are *Staphylococcus aureus* or Gram-negative organisms of faecal origin; between six months and two years of age *Staphylococcus aureus* and *Haemophilus influenzae* are predominant, and over two years of age *Staphylococcus aureus* is again the major cause. The insertion of artificial joints is associated with a slight risk of infection because the prostheses are made of plastic and metal, which are inert materials and which predispose to infection. Sources of infection may be the patient, the operating team or the theatre air. Late infection can occur and may be due to a transient bacteraemia.

Laboratory diagnosis. Blood cultures must be taken and synovial fluid should also be cultured. A primary site should be looked for and the appropriate material cultured. Synovial fluid appears turbid and creamy if infected, and will have a great increase in neutrophil polymorphs. (Exudate in rheumatoid arthritis looks turbid but no bacteria can be cultured.)

Treatment. This will be dictated by the organism isolated and the results of sensitivity testing. Aspiration of fluid is required and antibiotics are sometimes injected into the joint as well as administered systemically.

Osteomyelitis

Bacterial aetiology. This is generally an acute infection and is mostly caused by *Staphylococcus aureus.* Other bacteria that may be involved include *Streptococcus pneumoniae, Haemophilus, Salmonella, Brucella* and *Bacteroides* spp. The chronic condition may be caused by *Mycobacterium tuberculosis* especially in the Third World where it is a major cause of crippling disease with the spine or hip involved.

Pathogenesis and epidemiology. Any septic lesion in the body can be the source of the organisms and this

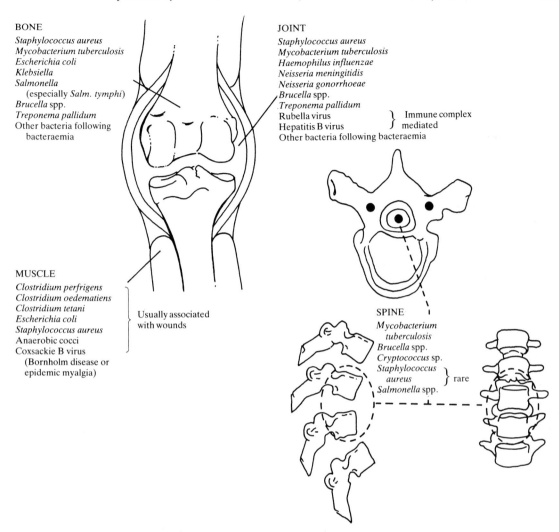

BONE

Staphylococcus aureus
Mycobacterium tuberculosis
Escherichia coli
Klebsiella
Salmonella
     (especially *Salm. tymphi*)
Brucella spp.
Treponema pallidum
Other bacteria following
     bacteraemia

JOINT

Staphylococcus aureus
Mycobacterium tuberculosis
Haemophilus influenzae
Neisseria meningitidis
Neisseria gonorrhoeae
Brucella spp.
Treponema pallidum
Rubella virus   } Immune complex
Hepatitis B virus } mediated
Other bacteria following bacteraemia

MUSCLE

Clostridium perfrigens
Clostridium oedematiens
Clostridium tetani
Escherichia coli
Staphylococcus aureus
Anaerobic cocci
Coxsackie B virus
     (Bornholm disease or
      epidemic myalgia)

Usually associated
with wounds

SPINE

Mycobacterium
     tuberculosis
Brucella spp.
Cryptococcus sp.
Staphylococcus
     aureus   } rare
Salmonella spp.

FIG. 18.2. Potential pathogens of muscle, bone and joint.

organism may be isolated from any collections of pus or fluid. In acute cases blood cultures may also be positive but rarely so in chronic osteomyelitis.

Osteomyelitis is uncommon in the jaws unless predisposing bone disease for example, Paget's disease or osteopetrosis, is present. Despite the frequency with which pus from a tooth abscess tracks into mandibular or maxillary bone, further infection other than that associated with the track of the abscess to the surface rarely occurs. The reasons for this are not clear.

The localised osteitis sometimes associated with tooth extraction (dry socket) is not an example of osteomyelitis but is caused by dissolution of the clot filling the socket. This condition is seen more frequently in molar sockets and often after extractions in which there has been some trauma to the socket. Infection of the clot by oral bacteria may be a factor. It is rare indeed for dry sockets to progress to osteomyelitis.

Treatment. Osteomyelitis is treated with drainage and the administration of antibiotics appropriate to the infecting organism. Penetration of infected bone is poor especially in chronic cases and for this reason antibiotics with good tissue penetration should be used. Before antibiotics are administered specimens should be sent to the laboratory for culture; pus, and pieces of necrotic bone are useful and blood cultures should be sent from cases of acute osteomyelitis.

Localised osteitis of the jaws (dry socket) should be treated locally with, for example, dextran powder and a covering of 'Orabase'. Antibiotics are rarely needed.

Gas gangrene

Bacterial aetiology. *Clostridium perfringens* is the organism involved in at least 60 per cent of cases. Others include *Clostridium oedematiens (novyi)*, *septicum*, *histolyticum* and the *bifermentans-sordellii* group.

Pathogenesis and epidemiology. Gas gangrene is caused by toxin production by clostridia and occurs when there is damaged or devitalised tissue which will provide the required conditions for anaerobic growth. The toxins cause tissue damage in addition to features of gas gangrene. *Clostridium perfrigens* and other clostridia can normally be isolated from faeces and their spores are ubiquitous in nature. They can be isolated from the skin of the perineum and thighs and when gas gangrene results from surgical intervention in these areas it is usually an endogenous infection. This type of infection is seen in older patients following mid-thigh amputations for ischaemic disease of the lower limbs. Three types of wound infection are recognised:

(1) simple contamination of wounds where the organisms do no harm, the commonest type of presentation.

(2) Clostridial cellulitis, an acute, spreading infection of the subcutaneous tissues.

(3) Clostridial myositis *or* true gas gangrene in which muscles are involved; septicaemia and toxaemia are common.

Laboratory diagnosis. Exudate or specimens of tissue should be examined. Gram-stained films will show large Gram-positive bacilli. Blood agar with and without an aminoglycoside should be incubated anaerobically. Biochemical reactions and toxin production should also be investigated.

Prophylaxis. Surgical removal of devitalised tissue is the basis of prophylaxis. When surgical procedures are to be carried out in the area of the thigh, perineum and buttocks, particularly in the elderly, prophylactic penicillin should be administered.

Treatment. Removal of devitalised tissue is again required as well as large doses of penicillin with or without metronidazole. In addition to polyvalent antitoxic serum hyperbaric oxygen therapy can be given to reduce anaerobiasis in affected tissues.

FURTHER READING

Adams E.B., Laurence D.R. & Smith J.W.G. (1969). *Tetanus*. Oxford, Blackwell Scientific Publications.
Christie A.B. (1980) *Infectious Diseases: Epidemiology and Clinical Practice*, 3rd Edition. Edinburgh, Churchill Livingstone.
Duguid J.P., Marmion B.P. & Swain R.H.A. (1978) *Mackie and McCartney, Medical Microbiology*, Vol. I. 13th Edition. Edinburgh, Churchill Livingstone.
Fallon R.J. (1979) Meningococcal diseases: pathogenesis and prevention. In *Recent Advances in Infection*. Reeves D. & Geddes A. Eds. Edinburgh, Churchill Livingstone.
Killey H.C., Seward G.R. & Kay L.W. (1975) *An Outline of Oral Surgery*. Part 1. Bristol, John Wright.

CHAPTER 19

Infections of the Liver and Gastrointestinal Tract

VIRAL HEPATITIS

A number of viruses are known to cause hepatitis especially in children, including cytomegalovirus and Epstein-Barr virus. The most important causes of viral hepatitis are Hepatitis A virus, Hepatitis B virus and the virus of non-A non-B hepatitis.

Hepatitis virus

Hepatitis A virus is an icosaherdral RNA virus with no envelope. It is relatively heat stable and is difficult to culture.

Hepatitis B virus has resisted all attempts at culture although electronmicroscopic and serological evidence have given some clues as to the nature of this virus. The complete infective particle, or Dane particle consists of a core of double-stranded DNA and a DNA polymerase. The capsid contains an antigen, the core antigen (HB_cAg); closely associiated with the nucleocapsid is the 'e' antigen (HB_eAg). Little is yet known about the HB_eAg although it appears in the patient's blood early in the disease and is regarded as a marker of infectivity. The lipoprotein surface coast of the virus is also an antigen, hepatitis B surface antigen - HB_sAg. Four major subtypes of HB_sAg are known. Serum from patients with hepatitis B infection contains many small spherical particles and some larger clindrical forms. These are thought to represent an over-abundant production of viral coat or surface antigen ($_sAg$). Occasional large spherical bodies represent the viron or Dane particle which contains all the components necessary for infection (Fig. 19.1). Hepatitis B virus particles are heat stable below 50°C and resist 100°C for a short time. Non-A non-B hepatitis is a serologically different disease from hepatitis B but no isolation of the virus has yet been reported. This condition probably represents infection by a number of viruses.

Epidemiology

There are many similarities between the types of hepatitis caused by these viruses. Differentiation of individual cases is on the basis of serological tests although the history of exposure may be helpful.

In hepatitis B infections particularly, cases may remain asymptomatic. Hepatitis A often occurs in epidemics associated with a poor standard of water supply but sporadic outbreaks can occur in institutions and from the consumption of molluscs. Hepatitis B infection is generally more severe, with some patients becoming carriers of developing chronic active hepatitis. The carriage of HB_sAg is 0.1–0.2 per cent for the U.K. and the U.S.A. but rises to two per cent in S. America, India and Russia and may be as high as 20 per cent in parts of Asia. N. Africa and E. Europe. Although most patients with hepatitis B infection recover and antibody (HB_sAb) appears, a few become carriers of HB_sAg and do not develop antibody. A very small proportion develop chronic active hepatitis and some develop hepatocellular carcinoma. Non-A non-B hepatitis resembles hepatitis B in many respects and is now the greatest cause of post-transfusion hepatitis. Screening of blood donors has largely removed the risk of transmitting hepatitis virus B by routine trnsfusion. Table 19.1 summarises the differences in laboratory findings and clinical appearance of these causes of viral hepatitis.

Hepatitis B infection

Hepatitis B surface antigen has been detected in many body fluids including blood, semen, saliva and

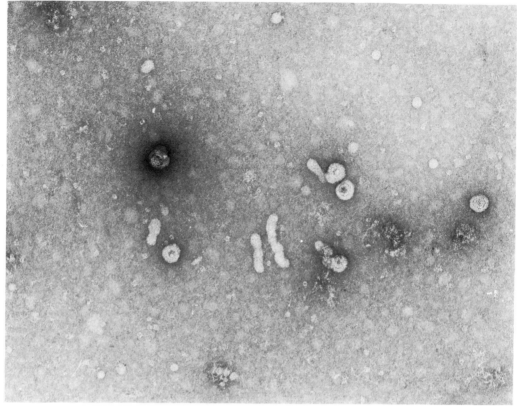

FIG. 19.1. Electronmicrograph of Hepatitis B virus in serum of a patient. This shows small particles (20nm) (HB$_s$Ag) and filaments (HB$_s$Ag). Dane particles or virions are also seen (45nm).

TABLE 19.1. Laboratory findings and clinical appearances in viral hepatitis.

	Hepatitis A	Hepatitis B	Non-A non-B hepatitis
Incubation	2–6 weeks	2–6 months	2 weeks–6 months
Onset	Acute	Usually insidious	Insidious
Age	Children	Any age but mostly adults	Any age but mostly adults
Seasonal onset	Autumn and Winter	None	None
Severity	Generally mild	More severe	More severe
Carrier state	Rare	Yes	Yes
Mortality	1%	1–40%	?
Fever	Common	Rare	?
Rash and arthralgia	Rare	Common	?
Transmission	Faecal-oral	Parenteral, venereal (especially among homosexual males)	Parenteral but may also be ingested
Detection of HB$_s$Ag in serum	No	Yes	No

urine. It is relatively easy to detect and is used as a marker of carriage of the virus, although it does not indicate that active infection is present. Once an HB$_s$Ag positive result has been obtained further tests can be carried out to determine the state of the disease in that particular patient. Full precautions can be taken with all clinical and laboratory procedures until the results of the further tests are known.

The appearance of antigen in the blood is followed by the development of specific antibody. Detection of these antigens and antibodies will help judge the state of the disease in the patient (Fig. 19.2). Tests to

women with active hepatitis B infection usually pass on the virus to the baby before or at delivery but symptomless carriers do not always transmit infection to their offspring.

The serious spread of hepatitis B infection in blood donations has now largely been eliminated following the introduction of screening procedures. In renal dialysis units infection has been particularly serious with patients, medical, nursing and laboratory staff contracting the disease. Careful screening of patients and specimens and strict laboratory procedures for at-risk specimens have been introduced to help eliminate the risk of such outbreaks in the future.

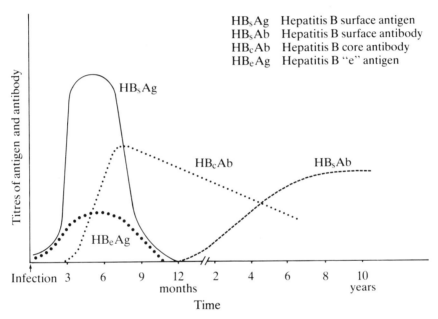

HB$_s$Ag	Hepatitis B surface antigen
HB$_s$Ab	Hepatitis B surface antibody
HB$_c$Ab	Hepatitis B core antibody
HB$_e$Ag	Hepatitis B "e" antigen

FIG. 19.2. Time course of appearance in serum of antigens of hepatitis B virus and antibodies to them.

detect antigen and antibody are usually performed by radioimmunoassay although less sensitive tests exist for screening for HB$_s$Ag. All specimens must be clearly marked for hepatitis testing and transported safely to the laboratory.

Although usually spread parenterally, non-parenteral spread of hepatitis B virus almost certainly occurs. There is, for example, a higher incidence of HB$_s$Ag positive patients among institutionalised subjects, patients with Down's syndrome, leukaemia, Hodgkin's disease and among male homosexuals. There is a strikingly high incidence of HB$_s$Ag positive patients among drug addicts and other cases where parenteral spread from unsterile needles is possible, for example, tattooing or acupuncture. Pregnant

Hepatitis B and the dentist

It is well known that hepatitis may spread by the parenteral transmission of small amounts of blood and that HB$_s$Ag at least is present in the saliva of healthy carriers. The risks in dental practice are:

(1) that the dentist or his staff contract the disease from a patient who is a carrier or is in the incubation period of the disease.

(2) that the dentist or his staff should pass on the disease to a patient.

(3) that the dentist could be involved in the transmission of the disease from one patient to another.

Evidence in the extensive literature on hepatitis in

dentistry supports all three statements. With an estimated carriage rate of 1 in 1000 in the U.K. it is calculated that 250 symptomless carriers are treated in a dental surgery every working day. Few of these will be known carriers. The incidence of HB$_s$Ag positive carriers among dentists is higher than in the general population and dentists have a higher incidence of the disease itself. In N Africa or parts of Asia, where the incidence of carriage is much greater, the corresponding risk to the dentist is greater. It is true, however, that the risk of a patient contracting hepatitis B from a dentist or *vice versa* remains small unless there is contact with fairly large amounts of blood, such as in oral surgery or periodontology. A number of recommendations have been made to improve the procedures in dental surgeries to minimise the risk of the spread of hepatitis. It is important to avoid the over-reaction of refusing dental treatment to patients known to be HB$_s$Ag positive. Most carriers will not be known and only in certain cases should extra precautions be taken and these usually in a hospital dental department. The recommendations of the British Expert Group on Hepatitis in Dentistry (Table 19.2) are simple to put into practice, require little change from current procedures and should be acceptable to dentist and patient alike.

The recommendations set out in Chapter 9 should be adequate for any dental surgery handling material contaminated with blood from a carrier. Routine use of such procedures should remove the risk to the dentist and staff of contracting hepatitis from the instruments. Disposable needles and sterile instruments should prevent the spread of hepatitis from one patient to another. It has been argued that dentists should wear disposable rubber gloves when treating all patients. This recommendation has found little support among practitioners who find operating in gloves reduces their sense of touch for delicate procedures. Clearly this measure would reduce considerably the risk of a dentist contracting hepatitis and it should be mandatory for oral surgeons and periodontologists to wear gloves when operating. This is not felt to be an encumbrance to other surgeons and there is evidence to show that practitioners in these two branches of dentistry are more likely to be HB$_s$Ag positive than other dentists.

Patients at Special Risk

The recommendations in Table 19.2 include a statement that patients at special risk should be treated in hospital dental departments. It is, however, perfectly possible for detailed serological tests to be carried out on such patients to determine their infectivity and those who are HB$_s$Ab positive whether or not they are HB$_s$Ag positive are safe to treat in general dental practice. Conversely, patients who are HB$_e$Ag positive are a particular infective risk and should only be treated with the sort of containment precautions that are possible in a hospital until they become HB$_s$Ab positive. It is worth noting that most patients with hepatitis recover and become perfectly safe to treat.

Procedure after exposure to infection

If a dentist or member of his staff comes into contact with contaminated blood it is important that they obtain anti-hepatitis B immunoglobulin as soon as possible and contact with the nearest Blood Transfusion Service, microbiology, Public Health Service or haematology laboratory should be made. It is sensible for all practitioners to be familiar with the procedure for hepatitis prophylaxis in their area.

The infected dentist

A dentist or a member of his staff closely involved in chairside procedures who becomes HB$_s$Ag positive should not be restricted unnecessarily from practice, but during any episode of active hepatitis should not work on patients. When the dentist or nurse has become HB$_s$Ab positive the infection risk disappears. At present the consensus of opinion is that even if a dentist does not become HB$_s$Ab. positive it is possible to carry on working with patients provided that gloves are worn in all cases. Several prospective studies have failed to show the transmission of hepatitis to patients from dentists who were chronic carriers of HB$_s$Ag and who had not developed HB$_s$Ab. In contrast it has been reported that 55 cases of serologically confirmed hepatitis B were traced to an oral surgeon who was HB$_s$Ag positive. When the surgeon began wearing gloves he stopped infecting patients long before he ceased to be a carrier.

Vaccination against Hepatitis B

Hepatitis B surface antigen (HB$_s$Ag) is produced in great excess during infection. Purified HB$_s$Ag preparations have been shown in animal and human studies to be effective vaccines against hepatitis B infection. The vaccine of HB$_s$Ag particles is not in itself infective but stimulates the production of antibody to HB$_s$Ag. Clinical trials have not reported any cases of hepatitis B infection occuring as a result of vaccination. Protection in animals lasts for about five years after which time a booster dose is required. Human trials have been under way since 1979 and commercially available vaccines are now in use. The

TABLE 19.2 Recommendations of the Expert Group on Hepatitis in Dentistry (1979), reproduced by kind permission of HMSO.

Patients who are known to be Symptomless Carriers of Hepatitis B Surface Antigen

(1) Those who are known to be symptomless carriers of hepatitis B surface antigen, and who are not in the special categories referred to in recommendation 4, may and should be treated in the general dental services provided reasonable precautions can be taken. These should include the following:

(a) The wearing of suitable gloves by dental surgeons and ancillary dental workers when working in the mouth, and by all surgery staff when cleaning instruments, benches or other surfaces, or preparing materials for sterilisation or disposal.

(b) The sterilisation (see Chapter 9) of all instruments that are to be re-used, including conventional low-speed handpieces (see g below).

(c) The use, wherever possible, of disposable instruments and dressings, which should preferably be incinerated after use or, failing this, sterilised and then discarded. Disposable instruments must never be re-used.

(d) The use of a fresh cartridge of local analgesic and a new disposable needle for each patient; this must be universal practice. Resterilisable needles must not be used.

(e) The wearing of spectacles (or eyeshield) and a facemask.

(f) The disinfection (see Chapter 9) of all working surfaces.

(g) The use of (a) conventional low-speed handpieces of a *sterilisable* type, and (b) traditional methods of scaling. High-speed handpieces and ultrasonic scalers can contribute to considerable splashing of blood and particulate matter which increases the risk of infection to the dentist and his staff.

(h) Wherever possible, known carriers should be treated at the end of a session.

(2) If these precautions are taken, all routine forms of dentistry, including surgical and conservative treatment, can be carried out with minimal risk.

(3) The use of similar precautions to those in (a) to (f) above when treating all patients would substantially reduce the small risk of contracting hepatitis from those symptomless carriers who have not been recognised as such; these constitute the majority of all carriers.

Special Categories of Patients

(4) The following are the main categories of patients, whether or not known to be HB$_s$Ag positive, who should be treated in hospital dental departments that have appropriate facilities. In certain circumstances these patients may present a higher risk of infection to dentists and their staff and many of them are known to be specially at risk of infection with hepatitis B.

(a) Patients with chronic renal failure who are receiving, or are likely to receive, regular dialysis treatment and patients who have had a renal or other organ transplant.

(b) Patients receiving long-term immunosuppressive therapy.

(c) Patients with haemophilia and others with haematological disorders who receive multiple transfusions of blood or blood products.

(d) Patients from institutions for the mentally handicapped. (Mentally handicapped patients living at home do not constitute a special risk)

(e) Known drug addicts.

(f) Patients suffering from jaundice which is thought to be infective in nature and those who have suffered from such jaundice within the previous six months.

---

vaccine is expensive but oral surgeons and periodontologists who, among dentists, are most exposed to patients' blood may consider vaccination worthwhile. Prior to vaccination it is necessary to check the subject for presence of HB$_s$Ag and antibody to HB$_s$Ag. Vaccination is given as two or three doses (depending on the particular vaccine used) and an antibody response can be demonstrated in approximately 95 per cent of recipients after this course.

THE GASTROINTESTINAL TRACT

Normal flora

The stomach and upper small intestine in both adults and children are generally sterile in Europeans, although in certain Eastern races, due presumably to different dietary habits, streptococci and lactobacilli may be present; in general diet has a major effect on gut flora. Once the ileum is reached a typical Gram-negative baccilary flora is seen, composed mainly of *Escherichia* coli and *Bacteroides*. The large intestine has a dense, varied flora, the composition of which is influenced by the distribution and composition of the intestinal contents, local defence mechanisms, physiolology of the host and diet. The organisms include *escherichia coli, Streptococcus faecalis, Bacteroides,* spp. *Lactobacillus* spp. *Clostridium* spp. anaerobic cocci. *Bifidobacterium* spp. *Klebsiella* spp. *Proteus* spp. and *Pseudomonas* spp.

Defences against infection (Table 19.3)

Potential pathogens (Fig. 19.4)

Various factors such as the size of the infecting dose, ability to adhere to and invade the gut and production of toxin influence whether or not infection is

TABLE 19.3. Defences against infection in the alimentary tract.

Dietary factors
Low pH of gastric juice
Lysozyme
Complement
Lactoferrin
Lymphokines
Intact normal flora
Local humoral mucosal antibody (secretory IgA)
IgG
Local cell-mediated immunity

---

produced in the gut. Normally the larger the challenge dose of organisms the greater is the likelihood of infection, as in cholera and brucellosis, but there are some gut infections that are associated with quite small numbers of bacteria, including bacillary dysentery, typhoid and infantile gastroenteritis caused by enteropathogenic strains of *Escherichia coli*. Viral infections may also produce symptoms.

Abscesses

These are an important form of sepsis and are

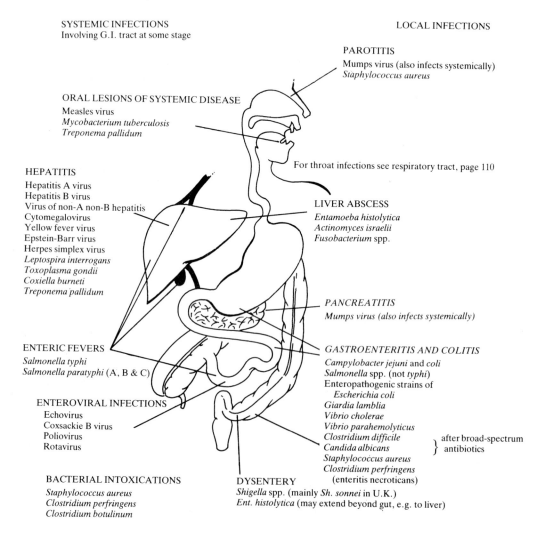

SYSTEMIC INFECTIONS
Involving G.I. tract at some stage

LOCAL INFECTIONS

PAROTITIS

Mumps virus (also infects systemically)
Staphylococcus aureus

ORAL LESIONS OF SYSTEMIC DISEASE

Measles virus
Mycobacterium tuberculosis
Treponema pallidum

For throat infections see respiratory tract, page 110

HEPATITIS

Hepatitis A virus
Hepatitis B virus
Virus of non-A non-B hepatitis
Cytomegalovirus
Yellow fever virus
Epstein-Barr virus
Herpes simplex virus
Leptospira interrogans
Toxoplasma gondii
Coxiella burneti
Treponema pallidum

LIVER ABSCESS

Entamoeba histolytica
Actinomyces israelii
Fusobacterium spp.

PANCREATITIS

Mumps virus (also infects systemically)

ENTERIC FEVERS

Salmonella typhi
Salmonella paratyphi (A, B & C)

GASTROENTERITIS AND COLITIS

Campylobacter jejuni and *coli*
Salmonella spp. (not *typhi*)
Enteropathogenic strains of
    Escherichia coli
Giardia lamblia
Vibrio cholerae
Vibrio parahemolyticus
Clostridium difficile   } after broad-spectrum
Candida albicans   } antibiotics
Staphylococcus aureus
Clostridium perfringens
(enteritis necroticans)

ENTEROVIRAL INFECTIONS

Echovirus
Coxsackie B virus
Poliovirus
Rotavirus

BACTERIAL INTOXICATIONS

Staphylococcus aureus
Clostridium perfringens
Clostridium botulinum

DYSENTERY

Shigella spp. (mainly *Sh. sonnei* in U.K.)
Ent. histolytica (may extend beyond gut, e.g. to liver)

N.B. a range of helminths can also infect the gastrointestinal tract

FIG. 19.3. Potential pathogens of gastrointestinal tract.

sometimes difficult to locate and diagnose. Because they are walled off by inflammatory reaction antibiotics alone are insufficient in treatment; surgical drainage is usually also required.

Abscesses may be clinically obvious (perianal and ischiorectal) or hidden (cryptogenic). The latter are difficult to diagnose and include the subphrenic, abdominal and pelvic types. Spread is commonly haematogenous; for example a liver abscess may be caused by bacteria carried in the portal vein from an abscess of the appendix.

Any component of the normal gut flora may be associated with liver or abdominal absecesses.

Brucellosis

Three main species of *Brucella* occur in different animal hosts:
(1) *Brucella abortus* : cattle,
(2) *Brucella melitensis* : sheep and goats, and
(3) *Brucella suis* : pigs.

Pathogenesis and epidemiology. Each of the species is pathogenic to man. *Brucella abortus* is the most common in the UK. Man is infected either by ingestion of unpasteurised milk from infected cows or goats or by handling infected animals or meat. Infection can be contracted through abrasions in the skin and through mucosae. Brucellosis has a world-wide distribution although it is classically associated with the Mediterranean littoral. It is an occupational hazard of butchers, veterinary surgeons and farmers.

Bacteria multiply inside macrophages and are resistant to killing by phagocytes.

Laboratory diagnosis. Repeated blood cultures should be taken; the organisms are difficult to culture and grow slowly. Serological tests are helpful from the second week of clinical infection, notably the complement fixation test and the direct and indirect agglutination tests.

Control. Eradication is favoured rather than vaccination in the UK. If antibodies to brucellae are detected in milk the animals are slaughtered.

Treatment. Cotrimoxazole or a combination of oral tetracycline and intramuscular strepromycin may be used.

Cholera

Bacterial aetiology. Two vibrios, the classical *Vibrio cholerae* and the *El Tor* biotype, cause cholera.

Pathogenesis and epidemiology. The source is usually a human case although symptomless carriers may also be involved.

Vibrios are ingested in food and water and surviving the acid barrier of the gastric juice begin to multiply in the intestinal contents, becoming attached to the epithelial cells of the small intestine. *Vibrio cholerae* organisms are non-invasive but as they multiply in the lumen they produce a powerful enterotoxin which activates adenyl cyclase, raising the concentration of cyclic AMP in cells. This results in an increased outpouring of water and electrolytes into the intestine and the effects of the disease such as severe dehydration are due to this. During the last twenty years *El Tor* has spread from the Far East to Southern Europe.

Cholera is highly communicable, transmitted from person to person via contaminated or un-cooked foods and water. During non-epidemic periods in endemic areas there is a high ratio of symptomless carriers to clinical cases particularly with the *El Tor* biotype, although explosive epidemics occur if a vehicle such as food or water is infected.

Laboratory diagnosis. A specimen of stool is examined for vibrios microscopically and also by culture.

Control. Separate sewage disposal systems and the provision of safe water supplies are vital. Control of cholera also includes isolation, treatment of infectious cases, surveillance of contracts and enforcement of proper community and group standards of hygiene. Prophylactic immunisation is not recommended because the available vaccines produce immunity that does not last longer than a few months.

Treatment. The most important treatment is to restore the vast loss of fluid and electrolytes. The mortality which can range from 50–70 per cent can be virtually abolished by this restoration of the acid-base balance. Later, tetracyclines may be given.

Dysentery

Bacterial aetiology

The genus *Shigella* contains four groups named *Shigella dysenteriae, flexneri, boydii* and *sonnei*. Bacillary dysentery is quite distinct from amoebic dysentery which is caused by *Entamoeba histolytica*.

Pathogenesis and epidemiology. Bacillary dysentery occurs by ingestion of the organisms. The bacilli attach themselves to the epithelial cells of the mucosal villi, enter these cells, multiply within them and spread into adjacent cells. The infected cells are killed and an inflammatory reaction results in the sub-mucosa and lamina propria with resulting necrosis and ulceration of the epithelium. Stools contain blood, pus and mucus. *Shigella dysenteriae* infection is usually imported into Europe and causes a particularly severe form of dysentery because of the production of a powerful enterotoxin, in addition to the lipopolysaccharide endotoxin formed by all *Shigella.* Unlike other *Shigella* infections *Shigella dysenteriae* infection may be life threatening. *Shigella flexneri* and *boydii* cause a less severe illness and *sonnei* infection which is the most common in the U.K. may only produce a few loose stools with slight abdominal discomfort.

In the main bacillary dysentery is spread from hand to mouth. A case or carrier can contaminate the hands at toilet and further contaminate door handles, lavatory chains and hand towels if personal hygiene is deficient. Subsequent handling of these by another person results in the transfer of the dysentery bacilli to the hands and possibly the mouth. Pre-school and primary school children are frequently involved in outbreaks of dysentery. Inadequate toilet facilities and the lack of attention to hand washing undoubtedly plays a part in the spread of the disease.

Laboratory diagnosis. A stool sample should be examined; this is much more satisfactory than a rectal swab. MacConkey and selective media such as desoxycholate citrate agar (DCA) are used for culture. Non-lactose fermenting colonies are then subjected to bio-chemical tests and identified serologically.

Prophylaxis. Attention to personal hygiene is very important but difficult to achieve in young children. The use of paper towels or hot air blowers rather than roller towels in institutions and the installation of washbasin taps operated by foot instead of by hand is recommended.

Treatment. Antibiotics have little part to play in this disease and may indeed prolong the period of excretion of the bacilli. An exception is in the treatment of *Shigella dysenteriae* infection for which cotrimoxazole, ampicillin or tetracyclines may be used.

Food poisoning

Bacterial food poisoning is an acute gastroenteritis resulting from ingesting contaminated food or drink. There are specific infections that can be transmitted by food and drink, such as typhoid, cholera, campylobacter gastroenteritis, brucellosis, Q fever and hepatitis, but the term 'food poisoning' does not embrace these.

Bacterial aetiology. Table 19.4 shows the types and percentage occurence of bacteria causing food poisoning in the UK in recent years.

TABLE 19.4. Percentage isolation of bacteria causing food poisoning in recent years from reports of the Public Health Laboratory Service.

Salmonella (particularly *typhimurium*)	80
Clostridium perfringens	15
Staphylococcus aureus	4
Escherichia coli	1–2
Bacillus cereus	0.5
Streptococcus faecalis *Vibrio parahaemolyticus* }	a few cases

Pathogenesis and epidemiology. Fig. 19.4 shows patterns of spread of infection.

There are three main types of poisoning:
(1) infective.
(2) toxic.
(3) toxic-infective.

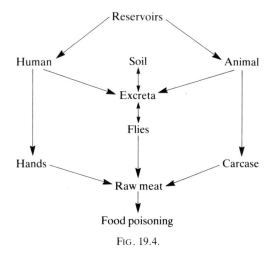

FIG. 19.4.

(1) *The infective type.* Salmonellae, other than those responsible for causing enteric fever, are the commonest causes of this form of food poisoning. There are over 700 species of these and many more serotypes. Important species include *typhimurium, newport, enteritidis, hadar, agona, heidelberg* and *panama.* The organisms multiply in the food and later in the intestine of the victim.

The 12-48 hours incubation period is longer than in toxic food poisoning and is followed by pyrexia and diarrhoea of one or two days' duration. Vomiting is not usually severe. Cold meats, sausages and occassionally eggs but particularly poultry are common sources of salmonellae. Bulk processing of food, intensive poultry farming and animal rearing have contributed greatly to the increasing incidence of food poisoning.

(2) *The toxic type.* This is most commonly produced by enterotoxigenic strains of *Staphylococcus aureus.* Staphylococcal food poisoning causes nausea, vomiting and often prostration with some diarrhoea within one to six hours of ingesting the contaminated food containing the pre-formed heat-stable toxin. Foods commonly incriminated include cream cakes, trifles, meat paste, pies and ham. The usual sources of staphylococci are the upper respiratory tract, particularly the nose, and septic lesions on the skin of food handlers.

Botulism. This follows ingestion of pre-formed toxin in food and drink and is often fatal. *Clostridium botulinum,* of which there are at least seven different serotypes, is the cause. The types associated with botulism in man, A and B, occur widely in soil, and type E is associated with fish. A potent neurotoxin is formed.

Bacillus cereus. This is associated with contaminated rice that has been kept warm after it has been cooked; the spores survive boiling. Symptoms are probably due to pre-formed enterotoxin. Two clinical types are described:

(1) staphylococcal-like, of rapid onset and with vomiting as the main feature, and

(2) clostridial-like, with a longer incubation period and with diarrhoea and abdominal pain.

Vibrio parahaemolyticus. The organism producing this type of food poisoning is a marine vibrio. It occurs throughout the world in coastal waters and is found in raw or inadequately cooked seafoods such as shellfish and crabmeat. The organism multiplies in the intestine and may produce a cholera-like enterotoxin. Patients usually suffer from vomiting, diarrhoea and abdominal pain.

(3) *The toxic-infective type.* Spores of *Clostridium perfringens* are widely distributed in nature. Many of these spores are heat resistant and survive the cooking process. Contaminated stews and meat are most commonly involved. During the cooling stage the organisms germinate and multiply in the meat reaching large numbers (10^7-10^8 per ml) in a few hours. The victim therefore ingests meat products containing millions of viable organisms. The clostridia sporulate in the gut and produce an enterotoxin.

Pre-cooked or bulk-cooked meat is usually involved and outbreaks often occur in schools, hospitals and canteens. The incubation period is around 12 hours and the main features of the disease are abdominal pains and diarrhoea. The summer is the commonest season for outbreaks because of high ambient temperatures and lack of refrigeration of prepared foods, allowing multiplication of organisms.

Laboratory diagnosis. Specimens of vomit, faeces and suspected foods should be analysed. *Clostridium perfringens* isolates should be serotyped.

Prophylaxis. Meat inspection, routine medical inspection of food handlers and education in matters of hygiene for all food handlers is mandatory. Hygienic premises, adequate cooking and prompt refrigeration of cooked food are essential. Raw and cooked meats must be kept separately.

Gastroenteritis and colitis

Campylobacter organisms, related to pathogenic vibrios, have been known as disease agents in animals for many years but it was not until the 1970s that they were recognised as major causes of acute human diarrhoeal disease.

Bacterial aetiology. Campylobacter coli and *jejuni.*

Pathogenesis and epidemiology. Any part of the small and large intestine may be affected. Dogs and cats have been reported as sources of infection but it is probable that mass-produced poultry could be the source and vehicle of infection. Raw milk has also been implicated. After recovery patients may become symptomless carriers.

Laboratory diagnosis. A specimen of stool should be cultured on selective media.

Treatment. This is a self-limiting infection but erythromycin is useful for relieving symptoms.

Infantile gastroenteritis

(1) *Due to Escherichia coli*

Bacterial aetiology. Specific serotypes such as 026, 055, 086, 0111, 0125, and many others are involved.

Pathogenesis and epidemiology. Children under two years of age and particularly bottle-fed babies may develop mild or severe diarrhoea that causes dehydration and may lead to death. The entero-pathogenicity of the strains of *Escherichia coli* that produce gastroenteritis is caused by an enterotoxin that has a cholera-like action on the intestine.

The disease nearly always occurs in maternity hospitals or neonatal wards.

Laboratory diagnosis. This is by serological identification of pink (lactose-fermenting) colonies growing on MacConkey's medium.

Treatment. Correction of fluid loss and electrolyte imbalance is required. Antibiotics are of no value.

(2) *Due to rotaviruses*

Gastroenteritis with diarrhoea is associated with rotaviruses, members of the reovirus group. Respiratory illness often accompanies the gastrointestinal upset. Older children and adults may also be affected and spread is common in the family.

Laboratory diagnosis. This is by electronmicroscopy of a specimen of stool or antigen detection by ELISA.

Treatment. Correction of fluid loss is required.

Travellers' diarrhoea

Polluted food or water may be responsible for this. Sufferers excrete enterotoxigenic strains of *Escherichia coli* that have a toxin similar to the cholera toxin.

Winter-vomiting disease

Caused by calici viruses symptoms range from mild to severe diarrhoea with vomiting. It is not confined to winter; outbreaks occur at any time of year and affect children and adults in institutions such as schools and hotels.

Yersinia diarrhoea

Yersinia pseudotuberculosis and *enterocolitica* can cause mild or severe diarrhoea, particularly in certain areas of Europe. It may be misdiagnosed as appendicitis since mesenteric adenitis is a common feature. The sources are wild and domestic animals and drinking contaminated water may be the route of spread.

Helminthic disease

Diarrhoea may be caused by tapeworms, roundworms and flukes. Spread of infection is usually anal-oral.

Protozoal diarrhoeal diseases

These include amoebic dysentery caused by *Entamoeba histolytica*, a hazard in the tropics and sub-tropics. Giardiasis caused by *Giardia lamblia* is an intestinal infection that is well recognised in the UK, Europe and Russia.

Pseudomembranous colitis

Diarrhoea is a common side effect of antibiotic therapy and is associated with oral tetracyclines, oral ampicillin and particularly oral clindamycin. In severe cases the colon has the appearance of a pseudo-membrane. Toxigenic strains of *Clostridium difficile* are considered to be responsible for the condition. The organism or its toxin may also be isolated from diarrhoea stools from patients who have not had antibiotics.

Enteric fever

Bacterial aetiology. The term enteric fever includes typhoid and paratyphoid infections and are caused by *Salmonella typhi* and *Salmonella paratyphi* A, B and C respectively.

Pathogenesis and epidemiology. Bacteraemia is the important feature of the illness and the bacilli are also present in large numbers in many organs. The pathogenicity of salmonellae appears to depend both on their ability to survive and grow inside macrophages and on the toxicity of their lipopolysaccharide O antigen. In addition, typhoid bacilli possess a glycolipid called the virulence (Vi) antigen which protects the microcapsule of the organism against phagocytosis and antibody.

The source of typhoid and paratyphoid infections is the human gut, either as a case or carrier and spread can be via water, food, or the faecal-oral routes. The most common cause of enteric fever in the U.K. is *Salmonella paratyphi B*.

After an attack of enteric fever the organisms may persist in the gall bladder and are excreted intermittently in the faeces.

Laboratory diagnosis. During the first seven to ten days blood culture is the examination of choice and in the second and third weeks stool cultures are usually positive; urine cultures may also be positive at this stage. A test for agglutinating antibody in serum, the Widal reaction, can be done in the second or third weeks but is of limited value as false positive results are common. Blood, stool and urine cultures are the most important tests and should be done repeatedly. Isolates are tested for sugar fermentation reactions and non-lactose fermenting colonies are subjected to further biochemical and serological tests.

Prophylaxis. Safer water supplies, adequate sewage disposal and attention to personal hygiene are of great importance. Bacteriological surveillance of workers in the food industry is essential. Immunisation is also possible.

Treatment. Chloramphenicol, ampicillin and cotrimoxazole are useful drugs both in the treatment of acute typhoid fever and of the carrier state.

FURTHER READING

Christie A.B. (1980) *Infectious Diseases; Epidemiology and Clinical Practice*, 3rd Edition. Edinburgh, Churchill Livingstone.

Collee J.G. (1974) Bacterial challenges in food. *Postgraduate Medical Journal*, **50**, 636–43.

Collee J.G. (1981) *Applied Medical Microbiology*, 2nd Edition. Oxford, Blackwell Scientific Publications.

Expert Group on Hepatitis in Dentistry (1979) London. HMSO.

Geddes A.M. (1973) Enteric fever, salmonellosis and food poisoning. *British Medical Journal*, **1**, 98–100.

Hobbs B.C. (1968) *Food Poisoning and Food Hygiene*. London, Arnold.

MacFarlane T.W. & Follett E.A.C. (1983) Hepatitis B vaccine. *British Dental Journal*, **154**, 39–41.

Rimland D. Parkin W.E. and Miller G.B. (1977) Hepatitis B outbreak traced to an oral surgeon. *New England Journal of Medicine*, **296**, 953–8.

Sims W. (1976) Serum hepatitis and the dental surgeon. *Journal of Dentistry*, **4**, 151–61.

Sims W. (1980) The problem of cross-infection in dental surgery with particular reference to serum hepatitis. *Journal of Dentistry*, **8**, 20–6.

CHAPTER 20

Infections of the Urinary and Genital Tracts

Normal flora of the urethra

Organisms are found in the distal part of the urethra and are most likely derived from the gut flora. These include *Escherichia coli*, *Proteus* spp, *Klebsiella* spp and *Pseudomonas* spp. various other coliform organisms, staphylococci, streptococci, lactobacilli and ureaplasmas (organisms resembling *Mycoplasma*).

Defences against infection

Bladder urine is normally sterile because of hydrokinetic and bactericidal mucosal factors. Hydrokinetic aspects include the dilution of residual urine in the bladder by inflow from the kidneys and the emptying of the bladder. The bactericidal mechanisms in the bladder mucosa cause a rapid clearing of bacteria from the mucosa, the mechanism of which is probably immunological. Local antibody, complement and lysozyme may be involved.

Potential pathogens (Fig. 20.1).

Normal flora of the vagina

Organisms are not uniformly distributed throughout the female genital tract. Some areas support growth of predominantly anaerobic flora whereas others support the growth of aerobes.

Many different species can be cultured from the vagina and surrounding areas. In general there are several groups of organisms commonly present: lactobacilli, diphtheroids, group B streptococci, anaerobic cocci, coliform organisms, *Streptococcus faecalis*, *Staphylococcus albus*, *Bacteroides* spp and

yeasts. However, because it is not fully known which organisms are pathogenic in the genital tract it is not possible to describe precisely what is the normal flora. There would seem to be considerable potential for endogenous infection.

Defences against infection in the female genital tract

Glycogen in the vaginal mucosa, controlled by the secretion of oestrogens and progesterone and acted upon by lactobacilli to produce lactic acid and an environment of pH 5, is important in the protection of the vagina in the newborn, whose hormones are derived from the mother, and in women in the reproductive age group. During childhood and after the menopause oestrogen activity is absent, glycogen is not deposited in the vaginal mucosa and the vaginal pH rises to between 6 and 7.

Vaginal and periurethral flora and intact epithelial surfaces also have a defensive role.

Potential pathogens (Fig. 20.2).

Sexually-transmitted diseases

Non-gonococcal urethritis (NGU)

Non-specific urethritis (NSU) is becoming increasingly replaced by the term non-gonococcal urethritis (NGU).

This is now the most common sexually transmitted disease in men and women. Although several organisms such as *Mycoplasma hominis* and *Trichomonas vaginalis* have been suggested as causative agents it seems likely that *Chlamydia trachomatis* is often the organism responsible, although ureaplasma

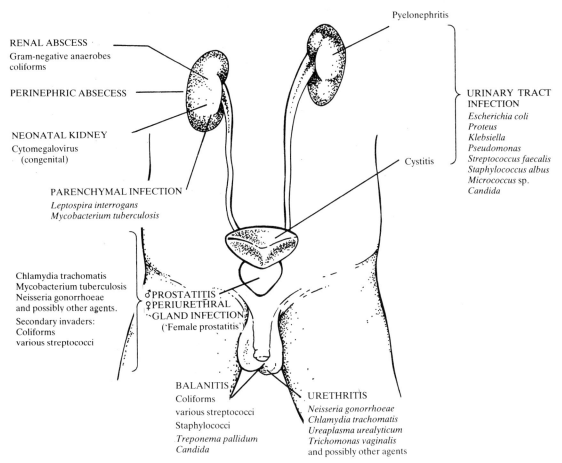

RENAL ABSCESS ·
Gram-negative anaerobes
coliforms

PERINEPHRIC ABSECESS

NEONATAL KIDNEY
Cytomegalovirus
(congenital)

PARENCHYMAL INFECTION
Leptospira interrogans
Mycobacterium tuberculosis

Pyelonephritis

URINARY TRACT
INFECTION
Escherichia coli
Proteus
Klebsiella
Pseudomonas
Streptococcus faecalis
Staphylococcus albus
Micrococcus sp.
Candida

Cystitis

Chlamydia trachomatis
Mycobacterium tuberculosis
Neisseria gonorrhoeae
and possibly other agents.
Secondary invaders:
Coliforms
various streptococci

♂PROSTATITIS
♀PERIURETHRAL
GLAND INFECTION
('Female prostatitis')

BALANITIS
Coliforms
various streptococci
Staphylococci
Treponema pallidum
Candida

URETHRITIS
Neisseria gonorrhoeae
Chlamydia trachomatis
Ureaplasma urealyticum
Trichomonas vaginalis
and possibly other agents

FIG. 20.1. Potential pathogens of the urinary system.

may be implicated in Chlamydia-negative NGU.

Laboratory diagnosis. Examination of urethral discharge and a first-catch specimen of urine will exclude the presence of gonococci. The presence of *Chlamydia trachomatis* can be identified by cell culture in McCoy cells using a urethral swab as the specimen. Micro-immunofluoresence monitors antibody production in infected patients.

Tetracyclines can be used to treat NSU/NGU, although not always with success because of its widely diverse aetiology.

Gonorrhoea

Bacterial aetiology. Neisseria gonorrhoeae (the gonococcus)

Pathogenesis and epidemiology. The gonococcus is a strictly human parasite. The anterior urethra is affected in men and the anterior urethra and cervix in women and infection is generally limited to the mucosa. Rectal infection occurs in both sexes and reports have described a 5-10 per cent carriage rate of gonococci in the throat. Gonococcal ophthalmia, an acute conjunctivitis in the newborn, may result from infection of the baby during birth.

Laboratory diagnosis. The best specimens from the female are a urethral and cervical swab. Vaginal swabs give inferior results. A swab of urethral discharge and of any discharge after prostatic massage is taken from males and rectal swabs may also be obtained. If possible cultures should be taken directly from the patient using a wire loop because the gonococcus is a delicate organism and dies quickly

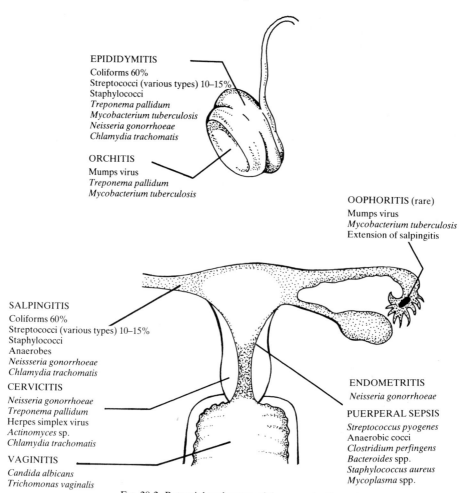

EPIDIDYMITIS

Coliforms 60%
Streptococci (various types) 10–15%
Staphylococci
Treponema pallidum
Mycobacterium tuberculosis
Neisseria gonorrhoeae
Chlamydia trachomatis

ORCHITIS

Mumps virus
Treponema pallidum
Mycobacterium tuberculosis

OOPHORITIS (rare)

Mumps virus
Mycobacterium tuberculosis
Extension of salpingitis

SALPINGITIS

Coliforms 60%
Streptococci (various types) 10–15%
Staphylococci
Anaerobes
Neisseria gonorrhoeae
Chlamydia trachomatis

CERVICITIS

Neisseria gonorrhoeae
Treponema pallidum
Herpes simplex virus
Actinomyces sp.
Chlamydia trachomatis

VAGINITIS

Candida albicans
Trichomonas vaginalis

ENDOMETRITIS

Neisseria gonorrhoeae

PUERPERAL SEPSIS

Streptococcus pyogenes
Anaerobic cocci
Clostridium perfingens
Bacteroides spp.
Staphylococcus aureus
Mycoplasma spp.

FIG. 20.2. Potential pathogens of the reproductive system.

outside the body; alternatively, transport media may be used. Highly nutrient laboratory media are required for its culture. Sugar fermentation tests and the oxidase test may be used to differentiate gonococci from other neisseriae.

In recent years many strains have been reported as penicillin resistant - partially or fully. Ampicillin is more effective than penicillin G or V for partially-resistant organisms. Spectinomycin and cefuroxime are effective for single-dose treatment of penicillin-resistant infections. Tetracycline and cotrimoxazole can be used but are less effective.

Syphilis

Bacterial aetiology. Treponema pallidum.

Pathogenesis and epidemiology. Almost all cases are contracted by sexual intercourse because like the gonococcus the causative organism is delicate and dies radpidly outside the body. The spirochaetes present in the superficial genital lesions are passed from one partner to another through intact or damaged mucosae. When the spirochaetes have established themselves at the point of entrance they multiply rapidly and within the next three months the 'primary sore' or 'chancre' appears, usually on the genitalia. This lasts for up to 14 days, then heals. Although the lesion is localised the spirochaetes are distributed widely throughout the body.

The secondary stage occurs six-eight weeks after exposure and lasts for three weeks - three months. Widespread skin rashes and other lesions may occur, such as the characteristic throat and mouth ulcers and condylomata of the anus and vulva. These mucosal lesions discharge large numbers of spirochaetes. About this time the primary chancre disappears leaving only a trace of its presence as a scar. The lesions of secondary syphilis are infectious.

The tertiary stage, the most destructive phase, is generally delayed for many years and takes the form of chronic granulomata known as gummata, in the brain, bone, heart, palate, skin and internal organs. Late manifestations of syphilis are degeneration of the brain cells producing general paralysis of the insane (GPI) and destruction of nerve fibres in the spinal cord causing tabes dorsalis. Lesions of tertiary syphilis contain few spirochaetes. The massive tissue damage may be accounted for by a delayed hypersensitivity reaction; no toxins have been described.

Laboratory diagnosis. This is either by demonstration of *Treponema pallidum*, by dark-ground microscopy (the organism cannot be grown on artificial media) or by serological tests, such as: (1) *Detection of antibodies against cardiolipin.* These include the Wassermann Reaction and Kahn test. These are non specific and false-positive reactions may occur. The Venereal Diseases Research Laboratory (VDRL) test is reliable and simple to perform.

(2) *Detection of anti-treponemal antibody.* The Reiter protein complement fixation (RPCF) test is a useful screening procedure.

(3) *Treponema pallidum (specific tests for).* The fluorescent treponemal antibody adsorbed (FTA-abs) test and the *Treponema pallidum* haemagglutination (TPHA) test are useful diagnostic procedures.

Penicillin is the drug of choice in treatment.

Trichomoniasis

A protozoal infection caused by *Trichomonas vaginalis*, this is a chronic infection of the vagina, characterised by a yellow, offensive discharge. Associated infection with *Neisseria gonorrhoeae* is not uncommon. Infection sometimes spreads to the urethra, cervix and Bartholin's glands.

Laboratory diagnosis. Examination of wet films of pus will reveal the characteristically motile *Trichomonas vaginalis* in cases of trichomonal vaginitis. Metronidazole is used in treatment.

Genital candidosis

Although several species of *Candida* can cause this the most common is *Candida albicans. Candida* may occur as commensal organisms in the vagina but they may also cause irritation, with a thick, white discharge. Infection is common in pregnancy and may follow broad-spectrum antibiotic therapy.

Laboratory diagnosis. A swab should be taken from the inflamed areas of the vagina. *Candida albicans* is usually quite easily found on Gram-stained films from the swab; Sabouraud's agar or malt agar plates should also be inoculated with the swab. Isolation of *Candida* does not necessarily imply infection but in a symptomatic case nystatin, amphotericin or imidazoles should be used in treatment.

In addition to the above several other infections can be transmitted sexually causing superficial lesions of the genitalia such as papules, vesicles and ulcers. These are:

(1) *Bacterial infections.*
Granuloma inguinale - *(Donovania* or *Calymmatobacterium granulomatis).*
Chancroid, 'soft sore' - *(Haemophilus ducreyi).*

(2) *Chlamydia trachomatis.*
Lymphogranuloma venereum.

(3) *Viruses.*
Herpes genitalis (Herpes simplex virus, usually type 2, but type 1 infection also occurs).
Warts (Papovavirus)
Molluscum contagiosum (pox virus)

(4) *Fungi*
Tinea cruris

(5) *Parasites*
Lice *(Phthirus pubis)*
Scabies *(Sarcoptes scabiei)*

Urinary tract infection (UTI)

Aetiology, Escherichia coli is responsible for the greatest number of cases, particularly serotypes 02, 04, 06 and 075, but *Proteus* and *Klebsiella* spp are also common. Coagulase-negative staphylococci are also prominent in causing infections, *Staphylococcus albus (epidermidis)* group 1 in women in hospital and *Micrococcus* group 3 in those outside hospital. *Streptococcus faecalis, Pseudomonas aeruginosa* and occasionally viruses, such as adenovirus, may be involved.

Pathogenesis and epidemiology. Although cystitis and pyelonephritis are the most common clinical manifestations of UTI, asymptomatic bacteriuria is the most common form of UTI. Up to 10 per cent of women have asymptomatic bacteriuria early in pregnancy and if untreated about half of these will develop acute UTI.

Frequency and dysuria are common symptoms especially in females of all ages. Infection spreads from the perineum, aided in females by the short distance between urethra and anus, the interposition of the vaginal introitus and the shortness of the urethra. Various factors contribute to this type of infection such as poor personal hygiene, mensstruation, sexual intercourse, pregnancy and in older women gynaecological problems such as prolapse and vaginitis.

In females recurrence of urinary tract infection is reasonably common due either to original treatment failure where an organism that has not been properly eradicated causes fresh infection or to a new bacterial strain.

Specimen collection. This is one of the most important areas in the investigation of a patient with UTI. Specimens must be free from contamination and sent promptly to the laboratory. If delay in transportation is anticipated they should be kept at 4°C. The following specimens can be obtained:

Midstream specimen (MSSU). The urethral meatus should be cleaned with water and females should separate the labia while passing urine.

Suprapubic aspiration of bladder urine. If it is difficult to collect an MSSU or previous findings have been equivocal it may be worthwhile to consider suprapubic aspiration. This should be used in infants.

Catheter specimens of urine should be submitted only if the catheter is already *in situ* because of the risk of introducing infection. The sample should be collected directly from the catheter and not from the collection bag.

Examination of MSSU

Microscopy. This is useful for detecting pus cells, epithelial cells, red blood cells and bacteria and should be performed on a centrifuged deposit. Both wet films and Gram-stained films may be examined.

Culture. Specimens are usually isolated on nutrient agar and MacConkey agar.

The number of organisms present in the specimen is an important indication of the presence of disease and these can be assessed in the laboratory by quantitative or semi-quantitative culture methods.

Bacterial counts. 10^5 organisms per ml of a single species represents a significant growth. Counts of 10^4 and less are of doubtful significance. Those between 10^4-10^5 per ml may or may not be significant and justify examination of a fresh specimen of urine.

Prophylaxis of UTI. This can be achieved by long-term administration of antibiotics usually in reduced dose to kill any organisms that enter the bladder from the gut but if this is done it is imperative to monitor closely and frequently the antibiotic sensitivity patterns of any organisms in the urine to detect any bacterial resistance. Where predisposing causes exist such as renal calculi or obstruction to the outflow of the bladder surgical intervention may be required.

Treatment of UTI. Antimicrobial treatment cannot be guessed at and a specimen of urine must be sent to the laboratory to ascertain:

(1) which organisms(s) may be implicated, and

(2) the antibiotic sensitivity patterns.

Drugs that are found useful in the treatment of UTI include the sulphonamides, nitrofurantoin and nalidixic acid for cystitis, and cotrimoxazole, ampicillin and the cephalosporins for pyelonephritis.

Glomerulonephritis

Aetiology. Numerous agents are known to be involved in this disease; these include tumours and various microorganisms, one of the most important of which is *Streptococcus pyogenes.* Many different serotypes can cause acute glomerulonephritis and the disease may follow streptococcal infection of the throat and skin. Pathogenic mechanisms include cross reactions between antibody to streptococcal antigens and glomerular basement membrane.

Laboratory diagnosis. Serological tests such as the estimation of the antistreptolysin O and antideoxyribonuclease B titres are more helpful than bacteriological tests.

Prophylaxis. Treatment of streptococcal throat infections is ineffective in preventing acute glomerulonephritis although treatment of skin lesions may have some benefit.

Antibiotics have no effect in the established disease.

Perinepheric abscess

This can arise:

(1) by extension of an abscess in the cortex of a kidney.

(2) by extension of an appendix abscess via periureteral lymphatics.

(3) from the blood.

Surgical drainage is mandatory.

Genitourinary tuberculosis

Tuberculosis of the kidney is a consequence of invasion of the blood by *Mycobacterium tuberculosis*. The epididymis and seminal vesticles may also become infected and tuberculous cystitis may occur. Treatment must be continued for up to two years using anti-tuberculous drugs.

Leptospirosis

Leptospires are widely distributed in nature and are all grouped as *Leptospira interrogans*, with subgroups such as *icterohaemorrhagiae* and *canicola*. They cause Weil's disease and canicola fever respectively. The organisms are excreted in the urine of brown rats and they gain entry to the host through abrasions or by drinking infected water. The kidney is the organ mostly affected. Penicillin is used in treatment but with limited success.

Balanitis

Infection of the prepuce can be caused by various microorganisms (Fig. 20.1).

Infections of the testes

Epididymitis

Infection occurs via the vas and is usually secondary to infection of the urinary tract, prostate and seminal vesicles. It can also occur after prostatectomy and urethral instrumentation.

The Gram-negative bacilli associated with urinary tract infection are frequently involved, and to a lesser extent staphylococci and gonococci. *Mycobacterium tuberculosis* and viruses are infrequent causes.

Culture of urine with consequent antimicrobial chemotherapy is essential.

Orchitis

This can occur either as an extension of epididymitis or via the bloodstream. It is a common manifestation of mumps and other viruses such as coxsackie may also be involved. *Treponema pallidum* may also be a cause.

Miscellaneous infections of the female genital tract

Vulvitis

This is commonly caused by *Trichomonas vaginalis* and yeasts but may be caused by gonococci.

Vulvovaginitis occurs in young girls often as the result of inadequate perineal hygiene but sometimes as a sequel to the presence of some foreign body in the vagina. Staphylococci and coliform organisms are often isolated.

Vaginitis

In addition to trichomonal and yeast infection a non-specific form of vaginitis occurs from which staphylococci, streptococci (groups A and B), coliform and other intestinal organisms may be isolated; this may be associated with the use of pessaries, douches and tampons.

Cervicitis

Acute cervicitis may be the result of injury during childbirth, or due to inflammatory lesions in the endometrium or vagina. Staphylococci, streptococci, coliform organisms, *Bacteroides* spp, as well as trichomonads and yeasts, may be involved. Acute cervicitis may also occur in sexually transmitted diseases such as gonorrhoea, chancroid and chlamydial infection.

Endometritis

Both the myometrium and pelvic peritoneum may be involved. This infection occurs most commonly following childbirth and abortions, and as the result of gonorrhoeal infection.

Salpingitis

Acute salpingitis may occur by upward spread of infection from the uterus, from the pelvic cellular tissue or from the bowel.

The ovaries are usually also involved (salpingo-oophoritis), the condition is commonly bilateral and there is frequently an associated pelvic peritonitis.

Pelvic inflammatory disease (PID)

Bacterial aetiology. *Neisseria gonorrhoeae*, coliforms and anaerobes such as *Bacteroides* and anaerobic cocci are involved.

Pathogenesis and epidemiology. This is a pelvic cellulitis usually combined with a pelvic peritonitis and can be a sequel of many of the infections of the female genital tract discussed above. It can complicate surgical operations on the uterus, fallopian tubes or ovaries and may be a consequence of infected bowel, uterine or cervical malignances.

Blood cultures should be taken and if laparotomy or laparoscopy is performed pus should be collected for examination. Vaginal swabs are unhelpful.

Puerperal sepsis

Bacterial aetiology. The most common organisms that affect the post-partum uterus are *Staphylococcus aureus*, beta-haemolytic streptococci, anaerobic cocci, *Bacteroides* spp and coliforms.

Pathogenesis and epidemiology. Puerperal sepsis is like a wound infection with consequent inflammatory reaction in the pelvic organs. Sources of infection may be exogenous or endogenous and before the days of proper aseptic technique was a considerable cause of maternal death.

Laboratory diagnosis. Cervical and high vaginal swabs may be useful but examination of pus or discharge is generally more helpful. Treatment will depend on the laboratory reports.

Genitourinary infection and the dentist

It is important that the dentist is aware of genitourinary infection because the pathological lesions produced by the sexually-transmitted diseases may also be present in the mouth and may be transmitted from patient to dentist.

Although syphilis is relatively uncommon in the U.K. this cannot be said for many areas in the world. Indeed it is endemic in some communities such as in the Eskimoes in Greenland.

Carriage of the gonococcus in the oral cavity is more common in male homosexuals and the dentist should be aware that the carriage of hepatitis B is also higher in this group.

Urinary tract infections do not impinge on dentistry except in so far as they represent a reason for the prescription of antibiotics to patients. This will result in changes in the oral flora and may affect the choice of antibiotics by the dentist should this be required in the course of dental treatment.

FURTHER READING

Cruickshank R., Duguid J.P., Marmion B.P. & Swain R.H.A. (1978) *Mackie and McCartney Medical Microbiology*, Vol. I, 13th Edition. Edinburgh, Churchill Livingstone.
O'Grady F. & Brumfitt W. (1968) *Urinary Tract Infection.* London, Oxford University Press.
Passmore R. & Robson J.S. (Eds.) (1980) *A Companion to Medical Studies*, Vol. 2, 2nd Edition. Oxford, Blackwell Scientific Publication.
Tyrrell D.A.J., Phillips I., Goodwin C.S. & Blowers R. (1980) *Microbial Disease: the use of the laboratory in diagnosis, therapy and control.* London: Edward Arnold.

CHAPTER 21

Infections of Wounds, Burns, Skin and Eye

Normal flora of skin

Many different species of bacteria may be found on the skin and it is convenient to divide these into 'transient' flora and 'normal' or 'resident' flora. A third category may exist — organisms that are essentially transient but which may multiply on the skin and remain there for a short time. Transient organisms are derived from the general environment and comprise an infinite variety of bacteria. They are only loosely attached to the skin by grease and other fats and can be removed easily by washing.

Resident organisms comprise a stable population in terms of numbers and composition and they are less easily removed from the skin than the transient organisms. The main components of the resident flora are staphylococci (mostly *Staphylococcus epidermidis* but also *Staphylococcus aureus,* particularly in hospital personnel), micrococci, propionibacteria and lipophilic, non-lipophilic and anaerobic diphtheroids. Some Gram-negative bacilli may be found but these are generally few in number.

Various areas of the body support different densities and species of bacteria and several factors are responsible for the ecological differences. These include temperature, humidity, hydration, availability of nutrients, hormonal influences and the effect of the free fatty acids and other bacterial inhibitors. In areas of greater moisture such as the axilla, perineum and scalp there is a greater density of organisms, whereas the low hydration of the *stratum corneum* prevents colonisation by transient bacteria.

Nutrients are derived from:

(1) fatty acids from sebaceous glands that form the greater part of the skin lipids.

(2) apocrine and eccrine sweat.

(3) the *stratum corneum* which contains amino acids and peptides.

The *stratum corneum*, the outermost layer of the epidermis, is around 15 cells thick and is a tough structure. Most organisms reside in the superficial layers. The remainder (20–30 per cent) reside in the deeper parts of the hair follicles where they are largely protected by lipids at the follicle mouths. There is evidence to show that they are not in the eccrine and apocrine glands or ducts.

The flora of the scalp (skin and hair) is different from that of other areas because of a rich sebaceous gland activity and because humidity is greater and temperature higher. Viridans streptococci, actinomycetes and coliform organisms can all be isolated from the scalp.

There are several methods that can be used for sampling bacteria on the skin. These are biopsy specimens, tapestripping, swabs, cylinder scrub, contact plate, velvet pad and agar syringe techniques.

Defences against infection

These include factors such as drying, intact skin, lysozyme in sweat, sebum and bacteriocins. Free fatty acids produced from hydrolysis of sebum triglycerides may be bactericidal or bacteriostatic.

Infection of wounds

Bacterial aetiology. Wound infection may be associated with many bacteria. *Staphylococcus aureus* and *Escherischia coli* are the dominant bacteria but outbreaks due to *Pseudomonas aeruginosa, Klebsiella aerogenes* and other Gram-negatives have been reported.

Serratia and beta-haemolytic streptococci are less commonly involved. Anaerobes such as *Clostri-*

TABLE 21.1

Potential pathogens of skin	Infection
BACTERIA	
Staphylococcus aureus	Bullous impetigo, Ritter's Disease (toxic epidermal necrolysis), folliculitis, breast abscess, furunculosis, carbuncle, ecthyma, sycosis barbae pustules, omphalitis.
Beta-haemolytic streptococcus	Impetigo, erysipelas, cellulitis, pemphigus.
Erysipelothrix rhusiopathiae	Erysipeloid
Propionibacterium acnes	Acne
Mycobacterium tuberculosis	Lupus vulgaris
Mycobacterium balnei	Swimming pool granuloma
Mycobacterium ulcerans	Cutaneous tuberculosis
Mycobacterium leprae	Leprosy
Bacillus anthracis	Anthrax (malignant pustule)
Actinomyces israelii	Actinomycosis
Haemophilus ducreyi	Chancroid
Treponemata	Syphilis, yaws, pinta
VIRUSES	
Herpes simplex	Cold sore, herpetic whitlow
Herpes zoster	Shingles, chickenpox
Papova virus	Common wart, plantar wart
Pox viruses	Molluscum contagiosum, orf, smallpox
Coxackie A virus	Hand, foot and mouth disease
FUNGI	
Candida albicans	Cutaneous candidosis and paronychia
Microsporum audouinii	Scalp ringworm (Tinea capitis)
Trichophyton rubrum	Tinea pedis and corporis
Epidermophyton floccosum	Tinea pedis and intertrigo
Trichophyton schoenleinii	Favus
Sporotrichum shenkii	Sporotrichosis
Cryptococcus neoformans	Cryptococcosis
Blastomyces dermatis *Paracoccidioides brasiliensis* }	Blastomycoses
PROTOZOA	
Leishmania tropica	Tropical sore
INFESTATIONS WITH INSECTS	
Sarcoptes scabiei	Scabies
Lice	Head, body, pubic region
Fleas	
Mites	Papular urticaria

Note: A number of infectious diseases have skin manifestations that are an integral part of the clinical picture.

dium, *Bacteroides* and anaerobic cocci may be found and frequently more than one bacterial species is isolated.

Pathogenesis and epidemiology. Infection can follow trauma, injections and bites but the most common type of infection is that following surgery. The source of infection is an infected case or a carrier and may be a member of staff or a patient. The reservoirs and vehicles of infection are legion but are in the main human skin, the environment and inanimate objects. Cross infection is produced by direct and indirect contact and by direct and indirect airborne routes.

Many factors influence the incidence of wound infection. Overcrowding in wards is important because opportunities for cross infection are greatly increased, because good aseptic techniques break down due to an adverse staff/patient ratio and because qualified staff do not have the time to monitor the wound infection rate. Generally speaking the shorter the pre- and postoperative stay in hospital the less are the chances of cross infection. The type of operation, its duration and the size of the wound play a role, as well as the general health of the patient; for example, diabetic patients have a higher sepsis rate then the average healthy person. Age is also important. Preoperative razor shaving can increase the risk of wound infection because of the trauma to the skin that this inevitably causes. Efficient cleansing of the wound site preoperatively and good postoperative wound care are essential in minimising risks of cross infection. Surveys in the U.K. have shown that wound sepsis is responsible for a mean excess stay of seven days in hospital.

Laboratory diagnosis. If pus is present this should be sent to the laboratory. If not, swabs or pieces of tissue should be sent.

Prophylaxis. This can be practised if there is a proper knowledge of sources, reservoirs and routes of infection. Sources are generally human and reservoirs are either human or inanimate. It is important to remember that transmission of organisms is more important from people than from the inanimate environment, such as non-sterile ward equipment, ward dust or bed linen. Ward and theatre practices must be constantly checked and appraised to ensure that aseptic techniques, sterilisation, nursing and medical procedures are sound. Bacteriological monitoring of theatre and ward staff on a regular basis is also recommended.

There is a place for chemoprophylaxis prior to and during operations, using narrow spectrum antibiotics, to protect against specific pathogens in high risk patients. For example, the risk of gas gangrene in patients with ischaemic limbs undergoing operations such as amputations through the thigh is almost eliminated by giving preoperative penicillin or erythromycin.

Management. When there is a sudden increase in postoperative wound infection, or if the general level is unacceptably high, bacteriological and epidemiological investigations must be instituted. Records must be kept and in this regard there should be a wound sepsis record book. This book should contain information relating to the numbers and names, ages and sex of infected patients, dates of admission, type of operation, onset of sepsis, names of theatre and ward staff and date of discharge from hospital, as well as organism(s) isolated, bacteriophage types (if

staphylococci) and antibiograms. Liaison with the laboratory is important and in this regard the appointment of an infection control officer, often a nursing sister, is essential.

Information gained from these records may (but not always) pinpoint the cause(s) of the increase in wound sepsis; for example, a member of staff who is a healthy carrier of the organism(s) responsible for infection, a breakdown in antiseptic or aseptic measures, faulty techniques, inadequate ventilation or overcrowding.

Infection of burns

Bacterial aetiology. Although almost any organisms invade a burn the most common are *Staphylococcus aureus, Pseudomonas aeruginosa,* other Gram-negative bacilli and beta-haemolytic streptococci. Most of these organisms do not greatly affect the healing of a burn or a graft except *Streptococcus pyogenes* which almost invariably cause grafts to fail. Infection is often mixed.

Pathogenesis and epidemiology. If a burn is not given specific prophylaxis it becomes colonised within 24 hours. Whereas colonisation may show no obvious pathological effects, it may lead to local sepsis with cellulitis in the tissues and to septicaemia. The necrotic surface of a burn is moist and provides a good culture medium where bacteria can multiply out of reach of the body's natural defences. Immunoglobulin levels are decreased for a few days after burning.

In a full-thickness burn, separation of the slough will take place in about three weeks; during this period Gram-negative bacilli are predominant. Later, when the slough separates Gram-positive organisms *Staphylococcus aureus* and perhaps *Streptococcus pyogenes* and micrococci are present in the largest numbers in the exposed granulation tissue.

Sources and routes of transmission of infection are much the same as for surgical wounds. Cross infection is more common than self infection and bacteria are transmitted to burns by contact with nurses' or other attendants' hands, by air from other patients or staff in the ward, by inanimate objects and by food.

Laboratory diagnosis. Burns should be swabbed for culture each time a dressing is changed. If there is evidence of superficial infection necrotic material in addition to swabs should be sent to the laboratory and if deep-tissue invasion or septicaemia is suspected blood cultures should be taken.

Prophylaxis. There is a high mortality rate in severe burns and because chemotherapy is often unsuccessful prophylaxis is of the utmost importance.

Proper surgical treatment is essential; the dead tissue is excised and the wound closed with split skin autografts, although this is not suitable for extensive burns which run the greatest risk of infection. These may be treated by delayed autografting after separation of slough.

Asepsis is important and dressings should be changed in an isolation room that has plenum (positive pressure) ventilation discharging to the outside.

Local antisepsis, or topical antimicrobial chemoprophylaxis, has been shown to reduce numbers of bacteria and subsequent infection. Compresses of 0.5 per cent silver nitrate are recommended (against *Pseudomonas),* as well as silver sulphadiazine cream, silver nitrate chlorhexidine cream and chlorhexidine cream (against *Staphylococcus aureus*).

Bacterial infections of the skin

Staphylococcal infections

The most common staphylococcal skin infection is the boil or furuncle, which is a typically circumscribed lesion with central suppuration. Pus eventually discharges and it heals leaving no scar.

A carbuncle is a large abscess that often occurs at the back of the neck in the thick collagenous tissues. It is a laterally-burrowing subcutaneous infection and there are multiple openings to the skin. Carbuncles may be single or multiple and commonly occur in diabetics. *Staphylococcus aureus* also causes breast abscess in nursing mothers, and other superficial lesions that include pustules, sycosis barbae (face), blepharitis (eyelid), stye (eyelash follicle), conjunctivitis and omphalitis (umbilical area). Ecthyma, bullous impetigo and toxic epidermal necrolysis are also caused by *Staphylococcus aureus.*

Streptococcal infections

Unlike staphylococcal infections of the skin that tend to remain localised, certain streptococcal infections such as cellulitis have a tendency to spread.

Streptococcus pyogenes is the beta-haemolytic streptococcus most commonly involved in skin infection. Erysipelas, a spreading infection of the dermis, is usually seen in elderly patients and lesions

can occur mostly on the face where the typical cheek-nose-cheek ('butterfly') rash is seen. Lesions also occur on the limbs. Impetigo is produced by *Streptococcus pyogenes* but tends to be less common than the staphylococcal form. Lesions are yellow and discrete and eventually form crusts. Scarlet fever is also associated with streptococcal infection, usually of the throat but occasionally as the result of wound infection.

Gram-negative infections

These infections are mostly associated with the moist areas of the skin such as the axilla, groin and perineum and are less common than the Gram-positive infections. Coliform organisms and anaerobes such as *Bacteroides* spp may be isolated from abscesses and *Proteus* spp are isolated from the axilla of persons who use underarm deodorants. *Pseudomonas aeruginosa* may be involved in chronic paronychia, often in association with *Candida* spp.

Viral infections of the skin

(1) Primary. These include *Herpes simplex virus,* type 1, that produces the chacteristic vesicular lesions (for example, 'cold sores' on lips), *Herpes zoster* (shingles) and papova viruses that cause warts. Pox viruses can produce molluscum contagiosum and orf. Coxackie A virus causes hand, foot and mouth disease.

(2) Associated with infectious diseases. Many specific infections have skin manifestations that are major features of the diseases. These include rubella, measles, chickenpox, smallpox, glandular fever and ECHO virus infections. Rashes may also be caused in septicaemic bacterial disease, for example, meningococcaemia, and in rickettsial infections (spotted fevers).

Diagnosis includes electronmicroscopy and tissue culture of a biopsy specimen, vesicular fluid or swab, as well as serology.

Miscellaneous skin infections

Acne

Bacterial aetiology. Propionibacterium acnes, . Staphylococcus epidermidis.

Pathogenesis. Acne vulgaris is not an infectious disease. It is a disorder of the pilosebaceous system and certain pathogenic mechanisms can be identified. These are:

(1) production of certain factors by the above bacteria which may produce inflammation (free fatty acids are important),

(2) a certain hormonal imbalance, particularly androgenic stimulation causing an increase in the size of sebaceous glands (there is a close correlation between the size of the sebaceous glands and the severity of acne), and

(3) the duct draining sebum from the gland to the skin surface may become blocked with keratin.

Anthrax

Bacterial aetiology. Bacillus anthracis.

Pathogenesis and epidemiology. This is primarily a disease of animals, particularly horses, cattle, sheep and goats. Infection in animals is the result of inhalation, or direct inoculation of spores or vegetative cells into breaches of the skin.

Human anthrax, which is uncommon, is associated with farmers, butchers and veterinary workers, in addition to those in industrial occupations who are in contact with diseased animals or their products, such as workers in woollen mills and tanneries. Products that may cause risk of anthrax include wool, skins, bone meal, hair and bristles.

Leprosy

Bacterial aetiology. Mycobacterium leprae.

Pathogenesis and epidemiology. Leprosy is a chronic granulomatous disease of humans. Animals cannot be infected, although experimental infection of the mouse foot-pad is possible. The lepromatous or nodular forms are due to a deficiency of cell-mediated immunity and the skin, mucosae, peripheral nerves and various organs may all be involved.

In the tuberculoid form there is infiltration of motor and sensory nerves.

There are around 12 million leprosy patients in developing countries. Spread of disease is probably by droplet infection although the level of infectivity is low and requires prolonged and close contact.

Laboratory diagnosis. Skin biopsy should be done and a section should be stained. *Mycobacterium leprae* are acid fast bacilli and these may be counted on the section.

Treatment. Antimicrobial agents such as dapsone, acedadapsone, rifampicin and clofazime can be used depending on the type and stage of the leprosy and the condition of the patient.

Fungal infections of the skin

These are caused by two main groups of organisms, the dermatophytes and *Candida albicans.* The dermatophytes *(Microsporum, Epidermophyton* and *Trichophyton),* derived from soil fungi, have adapted themselves to live a parasitic existence on the keratinised tissues of man and animals. They survive in the horny layer, hair and nail, as well as the keratin debris shed from the skin. Human infection is frequently contracted from infected scales shed in communal washing areas, showers and swimming pools.

Candida species are widely distributed in nature and *Candida albicans* is the organism most commonly pathogenic for man. It leads a saprophytic existence in the mouth, gut and vagina, from which sites spread to the mucosae and skin may occur if circumstances are favourable for their growth. These circumstances include altered hormonal balance such as pregnancy, metabolic diseases such as diabetes and steroid therapy or the administration of antibiotics, in general anything that compromise the host's immunological system or the local microbiological balance.

Diagnosis is based on microsocopic examination of a smear or biopsy when invading pseudohyphae may be seen. Culture of the yeast is often helpful and unlike the dermatophytes this takes only a few days.

Wound and skin infections and the dentist

The dentist must be aware of any contagious skin disease in his patients so that cross-infection can be avoided. Similarly dentists with skin infection, particularly of the hand, must take precautions to avoid transmitting this to their patients. The management of wounds and burns is relevant to all practitioners but especially to hospital dentists and oral surgeons. Oral wounds are not often troublesome although staphylococci from the nose of the surgeon can just as easily contaminate an oral wound as any other. Oral surgeons must adopt the rigorous measures to prevent wound infection that are commonly used by their surgical colleagues especially when the operation site includes facial skin.

Infections of the eye

Orbital cellulitis

Infection has usually spread from adjacent tissues

such as teeth and sinuses and the organisms involved are generally those relevant to these areas.

The lacrimal (lachrymal) apparatus

The lacrimal gland can be infected by local spread of organisms from nearby sites. Acute inflammation of the gland (dacryoadenitis) may also be associated with mumps and gonorrhoea. The lacrimal canaliculi may be similarly infected.

The eyelids

A stye is the commonest septic lesion of the eyelids and is an abscess in the follicle of an eyelash. *Staphylococcus aureus* is almost always the cause.

Acute conjunctivitis

If there is discharge which is purulent this usually indicates a bacterial infection. The organisms involved vary and include *Staphylococcus aureus, Haemophilus aegyptius* (Koch–Weeks bacillus), pneumococci, gonococci and meningococci. *Pseudomonas aeruginosa* may invade the conjuctiva after eye operations.

Mucopurulent conjunctivitis

This is an early sign of opthalmic herpes zoster. It can also be caused by *Chlamydia trachomatis* which produces a widespread infection in the tropics, trachoma, as well as simple conjunctivitis without involvement of the cornea — 'swimming-bath conjunctivitis'.

Nonpurulent conjunctivitis

This is commonly associated with viruses, notably adenoviruses types 1, 2, 3, 5, 6, 7a and 14. The conjunctivitis is often accompanied by other manifestations of adenovirus infection such as pharyngitis (pharyngo-conjunctival fever), lymphadenopathy or a vague febrile illness. Adenovirus type 8 causes a keratoconjunctivitis ('shipyard eye') in persons who have repeated corneal abrasion, due to dust, grit or metal particles. Herpes simplex virus may also cause primary and recurrent episodes of keratoconjunctivitis. In most cases of nonpurulent conjunctivitis, however, no microbial cause is identified.

Neonatal conjunctivitis

Organisms that produce conjunctivitis in adults can also do so in infants but the latter are additionally liable to infection from the mother's genital tract during labour. *'Ophthalmia neonatorum'* is defined in Britain as a purulent discharge from the eyes within three weeks of birth. Gonococci, chlamydiae, staphylococci, streptococci (group B), pseudomonads and coliforms may be involved.

Keratitis

Any infective causes of conjunctivitis can spread deeper to involve the cornea, causing ulcers or a spreading keratitis. Viruses such as herpes simplex, herpes zoster and vaccinia, bacteria such as pneumococci, gonococci and pseudomonads and fungi are associated with keratitis.

Endophthalmitis and panophthalmitis

Infections of the inner eye derive from infections of the outer eye, penetration of foreign bodies and infection during surgical operations.

Eye infections and the dentist

These happen more commonly to the dentist than to patients. Practitioners should ideally wear some form of eye protection to prevent or reduce the spray of bacteria and viruses into their eyes. Infectious particles are usually carried on the abrasive debris of tooth or amalgam and this adds to the risk. Transfer of staphylococci, virdans streptococci, and other bacteria, as well as yeasts, can cause infection this way. More seriously, herpes simplex virus can infect the eye and render the dentist susceptible to recurrrent herpetic infections of the eye (dendritic ulcers). Unusual infections may also occur such as those caused by the protozoon *Acanthamoeba*.

FURTHER READING

Christie A.B. (1980) *Infectious Diseases: Epidemiology and Clinical Practice.* 3rd Edition. Edinburgh, Churchill Livingstone.

Dubos R.J. & Hirsch J.G. (1965) *Bacterial and Mycotic Infections of Man,* 4th Edition. London, Pitman.

Duguid J.P., Marmion B.P. & Swain R.H.A. (1978) *Mackie and McCartney, Medical Microbiology,* 13th Edition, Vol. I. Edinburgh, Churchill Livingstone.

Gibson G.L. (1974) *Infection in hospital.* Edinburgh, Churchill Livingstone.

Lowbury E.J.L., Ayliffe G.A.J., Geddes A.M. & Williams J.D. (1975) *Control of Hospital Infection: A Practical Handbook.* London, Chapman and Hall.

Noble W.C. (1971) Microbial skin disease. *British Journal of Dermatology,* **86,** Suppl. 8.

Index